Essential Guide to Acute

...ter ca.
...s working

~e accepting th...
...e BMA Libra...
amped
...lled afte...

...hat you
...vise you

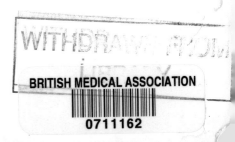

Essential Guide to Acute Care

Second edition

Nicola Cooper
Specialist Registrar in General Internal Medicine and Care of the Elderly
Yorkshire, UK

Kirsty Forrest
Consultant in Anaesthesia
The Leeds Teaching Hospitals NHS Trust, UK

Paul Cramp
Consultant in Anaesthesia and Intensive Care
Bradford Teaching Hospitals NHS Trust, UK

Blackwell
Publishing

Books

Blackwell Publishing, Inc., 350 Main Street, Malden, Massachusetts 02148-5020, USA
Blackwell Publishing Ltd, 9600 Garsington Road, Oxford OX4 2DQ, UK
Blackwell Publishing Asia Pty Ltd, 550 Swanston Street, Carlton, Victoria 3053, Australia

First published 2003
Second edition 2006

2 2007

Library of Congress Cataloging-in-Publication Data

Cooper, Nicola.
    Essential guide to acute care / Nicola Cooper, Kirsty Forrest, Paul
Cramp. — 2nd ed.
      p. ; cm.
    Includes bibliographical references and index.
    ISBN 978-1-4051-3972-4 (alk. paper)
    1. Critical care medicine.   I. Forrest, Kirsty. II. Cramp, Paul.
III. Title.
    [DNLM: 1. Critical Care.   WX 218 C777e 2006]
    RC86.7.C656 2006
    616.02′8–dc22   2006000965

ISBN 978-1-4051-3972-4

A catalogue record for this title is available from the British Library

Set in Charon Tec Ltd, Chennai, India, www.charontec.com
Printed and bound in India, by Replika Press Pvt. Ltd, Haryana

Commissioning Editor: Mary Banks
Editorial Assistant: Vicky Pittman
Development Editor: Vicki Donald
Production Controller: Debbie Wyer

For further information on Blackwell Publishing, visit our website:
www.blackwellpublishing.com

Contents

Foreword

The story behind this unique book started when one of the authors took up a post in intensive care medicine in order to learn how to deal with sick patients. It soon became apparent that almost everything learned in that post was immediately applicable to the general wards, both medical and surgical, and the Emergency Department. Sick patients are everywhere and it is a sad fact that even though doctors in the acute specialities deal with sick patients all the time, they often do not do it as well as they should. Awareness of acute care is thankfully increasing and one of the reasons for this change is because many people (the authors included) campaigned for acute care to be a core component of training for all doctors.

This book has been written out of a passion to explain in simple terms 'everything you really need to know but no one told you' about the recognition and management of a sick adult. Unlike most medical books, this one does not give you a list of things to do, nor does it bore you with small print. This book helps you understand what you need to do and why. The second edition has been extensively re-written and updated, with algorithms and references in a clear, simple format. The authors are medical educators as well as busy clinicians who envisage that this book will be used by teachers as well as learners. I recommend it highly.

Alastair McGowan OBE FRCP (Ed) FRCP (Lond) FRCS (Ed) FRCA FCEM
Consultant, Emergency Medicine
Immediate Past President, Faculty of Accident and Emergency Medicine, UK

Introduction

… in the beginning of the malady it is easy to cure but difficult to detect, but in the course of time, not having been either detected or treated … it becomes easy to detect but difficult to cure.' Niccolo Machiavelli, The Prince

This book is aimed at Foundation Programme trainees and for trainees in medicine, surgery, anaesthesia and emergency medicine – people who deal with acutely ill adults. Foundation Programme trainers, final year medical students and nursing staff working in critical care areas will also find this book extremely useful.

There are many books on the management of patients who are acutely ill, but all have a traditional 'recipe' format. One looks up a diagnosis, and the management is summarised. Few of us are trained how to deal with the generic altered physiology that accompanies acute illness. The result is that many doctors are unable to deal logically with patients in physiological decline and this often leads to suboptimal care.

In surveys of junior doctors of all specialities, few can explain how different oxygen masks work, the different reasons why $PaCO_2$ rises, what a fluid challenge is and how to treat organ failure effectively.

This book contains information you really need to know that is not found in standard textbooks. Throughout the text there are 'mini-tutorials' that explain the latest thinking or controversies. Case histories, key references and further reading are included at the end of each chapter. The second edition has been extensively re-written and updated. It is our aim that this book should provide a foundation in learning how to care effectively for acutely ill adults.

Nicola Cooper, Kirsty Forrest and Paul Cramp

Acknowledgements

The authors would like to thank their 'other halves', Robert Cooper, Derek Charleston and Gill Cramp, for their support in the writing of this book.

The authors would also like to thank those colleagues who gave helpful insight and criticism of the manuscript, and to all the medical students, nursing staff and junior doctors we have taught whose understanding and questions have shaped our writing.

Units used in this book

Standard international (SI) units are used throughout this book, with metric units in brackets wherever these differ. Below are some reference ranges for common blood results. Reference ranges vary from laboratory to laboratory.

Metric units $\times$ conversion factor = SI units.

Test	Metric units	Conversion factor	SI units
Sodium	135–145 meq/l	1	135–145 mmol/l
Potassium	3.5–5.0 meq/l	1	3.5–5.0 mmol/l
Urea (blood urea nitrogen)	8–20 mg/dl	0.36	2.9–7.1 mmol/l
Creatinine	0.6–1.2 mg/dl	83.3	50–100 μmol/l
Glucose	60–115 mg/dl	0.06	3.3–6.3 mmol/l
Partial pressure O_2	83–108 mmHg	0.13	11–14.36 kPa
Partial pressure CO_2	32–48 mmHg	0.13	4.26–6.38 kPa
Bicarbonate	22–28 meq/l	1	22–28 mmol/l
Calcium	8.5–10.5 mg/dl	0.25	2.1–2.6 mmol/l
Chloride	98–107 meq/l	1	98–107 mmol/l
Lactate	0.5–2.0 meq/l	1	0.5–2.0 mmol/l

CHAPTER 1
Patients at risk

By the end of this chapter you will be able to:

- Define resuscitation
- Understand the importance of the generic altered physiology that accompanies acute illness
- Know about national and international developments in this area
- Know how to assess and manage an acutely ill patient using the ABCDE system
- Understand the benefits and limitations of intensive care
- Know how to communicate effectively with colleagues about acutely ill patients
- Have a context for the chapters that follow

What is resuscitation?

When we talk about 'resuscitation' we often think of cardiopulmonary resuscitation (CPR), which is a significant part of healthcare training. International organisations govern resuscitation protocols. Yet survival to discharge after in-hospital CPR is poor, around 6% if the rhythm is non-shockable (the majority of cases). Public perception of CPR is informed by television which has far better outcomes than in reality [1].

A great deal of attention is focused on saving life after cardiac arrest. But the vast majority of in-hospital cardiac arrests are predictable. Until recently, hardly any attention was focused on detecting commonplace reversible physiological deterioration and in preventing cardiac arrest in the first place. However, there have been an increasing number of articles published on this subject. As a Lancet series on acute care observed, 'the greatest opportunity to improve outcomes for patients over the next quarter century will probably not come from discovering new treatments but from learning how to deliver existing effective therapies' [2].

In one study, 84% of patients had documented observations of clinical deterioration or new complaints within 8 h of cardiopulmonary arrest [3]; 70% had either deterioration in respiratory or mental function observed during this time. While there did not appear to be any single reproducible warning sign, the average respiratory rate of the patients prior to arrest was 30/min. The investigators observed that the predominantly respiratory and metabolic derangements which preceded cardiac arrest (hypoxaemia, hypotension and acidosis) were not rapidly fatal and that efforts to predict and prevent arrest would therefore be beneficial. Only 8% of patients survived to discharge after CPR. A subsequent similar study observed that documented physiological deterioration occurred within 6 h in 66% of patients with cardiac arrest, but effective action was often not taken [4].

Researchers have commented that there appears to be a failure of *systems* to recognise and effectively intervene when patients in hospital deteriorate. A frequently quoted study is that by McQuillan *et al.*, which looked at 100 consecutive emergency intensive care unit (ICU) admissions [5]. Two external assessors found that only 20 cases were well managed beforehand. The majority (54) received suboptimal care prior to admission to ICU and there was disagreement over the remaining 26 cases. The patients were of a similar case-mix and APACHE 2 scores (Acute Physiological and Chronic Health Evaluation). In the suboptimal group, ICU admission was considered late in 69% cases and avoidable in up to 41%. The main causes of suboptimal care were considered to be failure of organisation, lack of knowledge, failure to appreciate the clinical urgency, lack of supervision and failure to seek advice. Suboptimal care (failure to adequately manage the airway, oxygen therapy, breathing and circulation) was equally likely on a surgical or medical ward, and contributed to the subsequent mortality of one-third of patients. Hospital mortality was significantly increased in the patients who had received suboptimal care (56% vs 35%). The authors wrote: 'this ... suggests a fundamental problem of failure to appreciate that airway, breathing and circulation are the prerequisites of life and that their dysfunction are the common denominators of death'. Similar findings have been reported in other studies [6].

Following this, a number of other publications have showed that simple physiological observations identify high-risk hospital in-patients [7,8] and that implementing a system, whereby experienced staff are called when there are seriously abnormal vital signs, improves outcome and utilisation of intensive care resources [9–14].

Resuscitation is therefore not about CPR, but about recognising and effectively treating patients in physiological decline. This is an area of medicine that has been neglected in terms of training, organisation and resources. Some have begun to question the logic of a cardiac arrest team (when it is usually too late) and have begun to look at ways of better managing acutely ill patients in hospital.

Medical emergency teams

Medical emergency teams (METs) were developed in Australia and consist of doctors and nurses trained in advanced resuscitation skills. The idea is that seriously abnormal vital signs trigger an emergency call, rather than waiting for cardiopulmonary arrest. Box 1.1 shows the original MET calling criteria. In the UK, early warning scores have been developed to trigger emergency calls (see Fig. 1.1), usually to the patient's own team or the ICU outreach team, which is often nurse led. Up to 30% patients admitted to ICUs in the

Box 1.1 MET calling criteria

Airway
If threatened

Breathing
All respiratory arrests
Respiratory rate <5/min or >36/min

Circulation
All cardiac arrests
Pulse rate <40/min or >140/min
Systolic blood pressure <90 mmHg

Neurology
Sudden fall in level of consciousness
Repeated or extended seizures

Other
Any patient you are seriously worried about that does not fit the above
criteria

Reproduced with permission by Prof. Ken Hillman, University of New South Wales,
Division of Critical Care, Liverpool Hospital, Sydney, Australia.

Score	3	2	1	0	1	2	3
Heart rate		<40	41–50	51–100	101–110	111–130	>130
Systolic BP	<70	71–80	81–100	101–179	180–199	200–220	>220
Respiratory rate		<8	8–11	12–20	21–25	26–30	>30
Conscious level			New confusion	A	V	P	U
Urine (ml/4 h)	<80	80–120	120–200		>800		
O₂ saturations	<85%	86–89%	90–94%	>95%			
O₂ therapy	NIV or CPAP	>10 l RB or >60%	Any O₂ therapy				

Figure 1.1 An example of a modified early warning score (MEWS). Each observation
has a score: If the total score is 4 or more (the cut-off varies between institutions),
a doctor is called to assess the patient. If the score is 6 or more, or the patient fails
to improve after previous review, a senior doctor is called to assess the patient.
BP: blood pressure; NIV: non-invasive ventilation; CPAP: non-invasive continuous
positive airway pressure; RB: reservoir bag; A: alert; V: responds to verbal
commands; P: responds to painful stimuli and U: unresponsive.

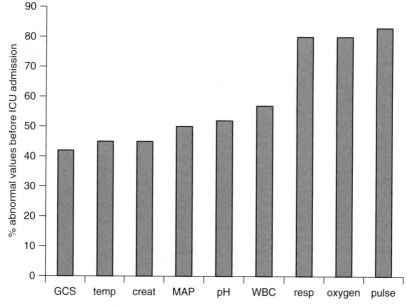

Figure 1.2 Percentage of patients with abnormal physiology in the 24 h preceding ICU admission. GCS: Glasgow Coma Score; temp: temperature; creat: creatinine; MAP: mean arterial blood pressure; WBC: white blood cells; resp: respiratory rate; oxygen: oxygen saturations and pulse: pulse rate. Reproduced with permission from Theta Press LTD. Goldhill D. Medical Emergency Teams. *Care of the Critically Ill* 2000; **16(6)**: 209–212.

UK have had a cardiac or respiratory arrest in the preceding 24 h. Most of these are already hospital in-patients. Half die immediately and mortality for the rest on ICU is at least 70%. The purpose of an MET instead of a cardiac arrest team is simple – early action saves lives. As one of the pioneers of resuscitation commented, 'the most sophisticated intensive care often becomes unnecessarily expensive terminal care when the pre-ICU system fails' [15].

Early experience in the UK suggests that an MET instead of a cardiac arrest team reduces ICU mortality and the number of cardiac arrests, partly through an increase in 'do not attempt CPR' orders [9]. Most patients admitted to ICU have obvious physiological derangements that have been observed by ward staff (see Fig. 1.2), but they may not know who to call, or the doctors they call may be inexperienced in dealing with critical illness.

In 1999, the publication in the UK of the Audit Commission's *Critical to Success – The Place of Efficient and Effective Critical Care Services Within the Acute Hospital* [16] re-emphasised the concept of the patient at risk – patients at risk of their condition deteriorating into a need for critical care. The report advocated better training of medical and nursing staff, early warning scoring systems and 'outreach' critical care. The Commission commented that intensive

Level 0	Patients whose needs can be met through normal ward care in an acute hospital
Level 1	Patients at risk of their condition deteriorating, or those recently relocated from higher levels of care, whose needs can be met on an acute ward with additional advice and support from the critical care team
Level 2	Patients requiring more detailed observation or intervention including support for a single failing organ system or post-operative care and those 'stepping down' from higher levels of care
Level 3	Patients requiring advanced respiratory support alone or basic respiratory support together with support of at least two organ systems. This level includes all complex patients requiring support for multi-organ failure

Figure 1.3 UK severity of illness classification. Level 2 is equivalent to HDU care and level 3 is equivalent to ICU care. Comprehensive Critical Care, Department of Health, UK, May 2000. Reproduced with permission from the Department of Health.

care is something that tends to happen within four walls, but that patients should not be defined by what bed they occupy, but by their severity of illness (see Fig. 1.3).

Following this, *Comprehensive Critical Care – A Review of Adult Critical Care Services* [17] was published by the Department of Health. This report re-iterated the idea that patients should be classified according to their severity of illness and the necessary resources mobilised. With this report came funding for critical care outreach teams and an expansion in critical care beds. In the USA and parts of Europe, there is considerable provision of high-dependency units (HDUs). In most UK hospitals, it is recognised that there are not enough HDU-type facilities. A needs assessment survey in Wales, using objective criteria for HDU and ICU admission, found that 56% of these patients were being cared for on general wards rather than in critical care areas [18]. A 1-month needs assessment in Newcastle, UK found that 26% of the unselected emergency patients admitted to a medical admissions unit required a higher level of care; 17% needed level 1 care, 9% needed level 2 care and 0.5% needed level 3 care [19]. This would indicate the need for far more level 1–2 facilities in the UK than at present.

Although there are many different variations of early warning scores in use, it is probably the recognition of abnormal physiology, however measured, and a protocol that requires inexperienced staff to call for help that makes a difference, rather than the score itself. Patients at particular risk are recent emergency admissions, after major surgery and following discharge from intensive care.

The MERIT study

Although small studies in the UK, usually using historical controls, have shown improvements in outcome following the introduction of early warning scores and protocols, only one large-scale randomised controlled trial has been completed to date [20]. The Medical Early Response Intervention and Therapy (MERIT) study randomised 23 hospitals in Australia to either continue functioning as usual or to introduce a MET system, which included staff education, the introduction of MET calling criteria, raising awareness of the dangers of abnormal vital signs and the immediate availability of a MET. Introducing a MET system increased the number of emergency calls but did not appear to affect outcome. However, there may be a number of reasons why this negative result was reported:

- Cardiac arrest teams operated as a MET to some extent in the control hospitals, with half the calls to cardiac arrest teams in the control hospitals made without a cardiac arrest (compared with 80% in the MET system hospitals). This is in contrast to most UK hospitals where cardiac arrest teams are only called for suspected cardiac arrests.
- The rate of MET calls preceding unplanned ICU admission and unexpected deaths was low even when MET calling criteria were present, suggesting that the system was not fully implemented.
- Direct calls to ICU for assistance were not recorded.
- A reduction in cardiac arrests and unexpected deaths was seen in both the groups, possibly because the MET system was publicised in the Australian media during the study.

The investigators point out that similar complex interventions such as the introduction of trauma teams have taken up to 10 years before any effect on mortality has been detected, and we cannot ignore all the previous studies which have shown that a MET-type system reduces the incidence of unplanned ICU admissions, cardiopulmonary arrests and hospital mortality, albeit using historical controls. Given that there is overwhelming evidence that seriously ill patients receive inadequate care worldwide, and given that simple measures can reverse physiological decline if administered early, it would be difficult to ignore what is intuitively a 'good idea'.

NCEPOD report: an acute problem?

In 2005, the National Confidential Enquiry into Patient Outcome and Death (NCEPOD) published a report looking at the care of severely ill medical patients across UK hospitals [21]. The foreword to this report commented on the changes to working hours and postgraduate medical education that have taken place, leading to less experienced and overstretched junior doctors managing an increasingly complex in-patient load. This enquiry looked at medical patients referred to general ICUs across 226 hospitals (1677 patients). The median age of these patients was 60 years, but the mode was 70–80 years; 43% of patients were referred directly from accident and emergency departments and 34% from general wards. The most common indication was a respiratory problem, followed by cardiovascular, then neurological. The patients had a wide range of early warning scores, from 0 to 12 (mode 5). In 10% of cases the pre-ICU history and examination was deemed by external assessors to be unacceptable or incomplete. Only 58% of patients received both prompt and appropriate care. Inappropriately low oxygen concentrations and delayed fluid administration were common examples of suboptimal care. Record-keeping was poor, there was a lack of clear instructions given to nursing staff and vital signs were often inadequately recorded; 66% of patients had 'gross' physiological instability for at least 12 h before referral to ICU. Consultant physicians had no knowledge or input into 57% of referrals. CPR status was documented in only 10% of critically ill patients. The report re-iterates the themes of failure to seek advice, lack of supervision, failure to document vital signs and failure to appreciate the clinical urgency of seriously abnormal physiology.

ABCDE: an overview

History, examination, differential diagnosis and treatment will not immediately help someone who is critically ill. Diagnosis is irrelevant when the things that kill first are literally A (airway compromise), B (breathing problems) and C (circulation problems) – in that order. What the patient needs is resuscitation not deliberation. Patients can be alert and 'look' well from the end of the bed, but the clue is often in objective vital signs. Box 1.2 summarises the physiological and biochemical markers of severe illness. A common theme in studies is the inability of hospital staff to recognise when a patient is at risk of deterioration, even when these abnormalities are documented.

The most common abnormalities before cardiac arrest are hypoxaemia with an increased respiratory rate and hypotension leading to hypoperfusion with an accompanying metabolic acidosis and tissue hypoxia. If this is left untreated, a downward physiological spiral ensues. With time, these abnormalities may become resistant to treatment with fluids and drugs. Therefore early action is vital. The following chapters teach the theory behind ABCD in detail. Practical courses also exist which use scenario-based teaching on how to manage patients at risk (see Further resources). These are recommended because the ABC approach described below requires practical skills (e.g. assessment and management of the airway) which cannot be learned adequately from a book.

Box 1.2 Markers of severe illness

Physiological
Signs of massive sympathetic activation (e.g. tachycardia, hypertension, pale, shutdown)
Signs of systemic inflammation (see Chapter 6)
Signs of organ hypoperfusion (see Chapter 5)

Biochemical
Metabolic (lactic) acidosis
High or low white cell count
Low platelets
High creatinine
High C-reactive protein (CRP)

ABCDE is the initial approach to any patient who is acutely ill:
- A: assess *airway* and treat if needed.
- B: assess *breathing* and treat if needed.
- C: assess *circulation* and treat if needed.
- D: assess *disability* and treat if needed.
- E: *expose and examine* patient fully once A, B, C and D are stable. Further information gathering and tests can be done at this stage.
- *Do not move on* without treating an abnormality. For example, there is no point in doing arterial blood gases on a patient with an airway obstruction.

A more detailed version of the ABCDE system is shown in Box 1.3.

Patients with serious abnormal vital signs are an emergency. The management of such patients requires pro-activity, a sense of urgency and the continuous presence of the attending doctor. For example, if a patient is hypotensive and hypoxaemic from pneumonia, it is not acceptable for oxygen, fluids and antibiotics simply to be prescribed. The oxygen concentration may need to be changed several times before the PaO_2 is acceptable. More than one fluid challenge may be required to get an acceptable blood pressure – and even then, vasopressors may be needed if the patient remains hypotensive due to severe sepsis. Intravenous antibiotics need to be given immediately. ICU and CPR decisions need to be made at this time – not later. The emphasis is on both rapid and effective intervention.

Integral to the management of the acutely ill patient is the administration of effective analgesia. This is extremely important to the patient but also has a range of physiological benefits and is discussed further in Chapter 10.

Special considerations in the elderly

The proportion of older people is growing, especially the very old (over 85 years); 80% of people over 80 years function well and relatively independently. Only 1 in 20 elderly people live in institutions [22]. Since many acutely ill patients in hospital are elderly, it is important that healthcare staff understand that there are important differences in the physiology of elderly people. This in turn means that the interpretation of vital signs and the management of acute illness may be different.

The following are important physiological differences in the elderly:
- Reduced homeostatic reserve. Ageing is associated with a decline in organ function with a reduced ability to compensate. The following are reduced: normal PaO_2, cerebral blood flow, maximum heart rate and cardiac reserve, maximum oxygen consumption, renal blood flow, maximum urinary concentration, sodium and water homeostasis.
- Impaired immunity. Elderly patients commonly do not have a fever or raised white cell count in sepsis. Hypothermia may occur instead. A rigid abdomen is uncommon in the elderly with an 'acute abdomen' – they are likely to have a soft, but generally tender abdomen despite perforation, ischaemia or peritonitis.
- Different pharmacokinetics and pharmacodynamics. Iatrogenic disease is more common in the elderly.

Box 1.3 The ABCDE system

Airway
Examine for signs of upper airway obstruction
If necessary, do a head tilt-chin lift manoeuvre
Suction (only what you can see)
Simple airway adjuncts may be needed
Give high-concentration oxygen (see Chapter 2 for more details)

Breathing
Look at the chest
Assess rate, depth and symmetry of movement
Measure SpO_2
Quickly listen with a stethoscope (for air entry, wheeze and crackles)
You may need to use a bag and mask if the patient has inadequate
   ventilation
Treat wheeze, pneumothorax, fluid, collapse, infection, etc. (Is a
physiotherapist needed?)

Circulation
Assess limb temperature, capillary refill time, blood pressure, pulse and
   urine output
Insert a large bore cannula and send blood for tests
Give a fluid challenge if needed (see Chapter 5 for more details)

Disability
Make a note of the AVPU scale (*a*lert, responds to *v*oice, responds to
   *p*ain, *u*nresponsive)
Check pupil size and reactivity
Measure capillary glucose

Examination and planning
Are ABCD stable? If not, go back to the top and call for help
Complete any relevant examination (e.g. heart sounds, abdomen, full
   neurological exam)
Treat pain
Gather information from notes, charts and eyewitnesses
Do tests (e.g. arterial blood gases, X-rays, ECG, etc.)
Do not move an unstable patient without the right monitoring
   equipment and staff
Make ICU and CPR decisions
You should have called a senior colleague by now, if you have not done
   so already

- Common acute illnesses present atypically (e.g. with confusion or falls).
- Quiescent diseases are exacerbated by acute illness (e.g. heart failure may occur in pneumonia, old neurological signs may become pronounced in sepsis).
- Some clinical findings are not necessarily pathological in the elderly, (e.g. neck stiffness, a positive urine dipstick (in women), a few bilateral basal crackles in the lungs and reduced skin turgor).

Despite physiological differences, dysfunction in the elderly is always associated with disease, not ageing. But their impaired homeostatic reserve means that intervention is required earlier if it is to be successful. This is an important difference compared with young adults. Clinical decision-making should be made on an individual basis and never on the grounds of age alone. However, one has to balance the right to high-quality care without age discrimination with the wisdom to avoid aggressive but ultimately futile interventions. Involving a geriatrician in difficult decision-making is often helpful.

The benefits and limitations of intensive care

Physiological derangement and the need for admission to ICU are not the same. It would not be in the best interests of all patients to be admitted to an ICU. Instead optimising ward care or even palliative care may be required. This decision is based on evidence about prognosis, clinical experience (e.g. recognising when someone is dying) and takes in to account any expressed wishes of the patient. Intensive (level 3) care supports failing organ systems when there is potentially reversible disease. It is appropriate for patients requiring advanced respiratory support alone or support of at least two failing organ systems. High-dependency (level 2) care is appropriate for patients requiring detailed observation or intervention for a single failing organ system.

For the majority of healthcare workers who have never worked in an ICU, the benefits and limitations of what is available may be poorly understood. Patients with acute reversible disease benefit most from intensive care if they are admitted sooner rather than later. Waiting for someone to become even more seriously ill before contacting the ICU team does not make physiological sense and is not evidence-based. On the other hand, admission to ICU does not guarantee a successful outcome. Some patients may be so ill that they are unlikely to recover at all, even with intensive organ support. The overall mortality of patients admitted to ICU is around 25%. All potential admissions should therefore be assessed by an experienced doctor. Patients who are not admitted to intensive care should have a clear plan and their ward care optimised.

Communication and the critically ill

Healthcare is a high-risk industry. It has been estimated that the risk of dying due to an adverse event is nearly 1 in 100 for hospital in-patients [23]. In recent years 'patient safety' has become high profile, as medicine has started to learn from other industries such as nuclear power and aviation. Since healthcare is complex, there are many facets to patient safety. One important facet is known as 'human factors' – how people interact with each other and technology. Attitudes, good communication, teamwork and situation awareness are as important in managing an acutely ill patient as a good medical management plan, and unfortunately this is something that most of us have not been trained in. This is discussed in more detail in our companion book *Essential Guide to Generic Skills* [24].

A new doctor once asked his senior how to treat a patient who had had too much beta blocker. The senior was half listening, writing in some notes. Another senior was nearby and asked, 'What do you mean? – What is the pulse and blood pressure?' The new doctor replied, 'Pulse 30, blood pressure unrecordable'. Both seniors dashed to the patient's bedside. Good communication is important. Below is a simple system to follow when communicating about a seriously ill patient with colleagues, particularly over the phone.

Use the following structure:

1 State where you are and your request (e.g. 'Can you come to …').
2 Give a brief history (e.g. 'New admission with asthma').
3 Describe the vital signs (conscious level, pulse, blood pressure, respiratory rate, oxygen therapy and saturations, and urine output if relevant).

Further details can follow if needed. Summarising the vital signs is the only way to give the listener a sense of how urgent the situation is. Your colleague may have heard all he needs to know and be on his way. Or he may want to go through some more details and test results first. Either way, it is important to communicate clearly what help is required, particularly if you want your colleague to come and see the patient. The senior resident doctor (usually the Specialist Registrar in the UK) should always be informed about any seriously ill patient, *whether or not* his expertise is required.

The following chapters describe the theory behind the assessment and management of acutely ill adults. They are intended as a foundation on which experience and practical training can be built. Understanding and practising

---

Key points: patients at risk

- Resuscitation is about recognising and effectively intervening when patients have seriously abnormal vital signs.
- There is a wealth of research to show that our current systems fail when hospital in-patients deteriorate.
- Early effective intervention can improve outcome and utilisation of intensive care resources.
- Physiological derangement and the need for admission to ICU is not the same thing. All patients should be assessed by an experienced senior doctor.
- In order to communicate clearly to colleagues about acutely ill patients, use a simple system: what you want, brief history and a summary of the vital signs.
- Always inform the senior resident doctor about a seriously ill patient.

the basics well is the essence of good acute care, which can even be summed up as 'the right oxygen, the right fluid and the right help at the right time'. We hope that by the end of this book, you will have a better idea of what this means and have a better understanding of the significance of common clinical findings. These simple things can make a big difference to your patients.

References

1. Diem SJ, Lantos JD and Tulsky JA. Cardiopulmonary resuscitation on television. Miracles and misinformation. *New England Journal of Medicine* 1996; **334**: 1578–1582.
2. Pronovost PJ, Nolan T, Zeger S, Miller M and Rubin H. How can clinicians measure safety and quality in acute care? Inpatient safety ll. *Lancet* 2005; **363**: 1061–1067.
3. Schein RM, Hazday N, Pena N and Ruben BH. Clinical antecedents to in-hospital cardiopulmonary arrest. *Chest* 1990; **98**: 1388–1392.
4. Franklin C and Matthew J. Developing strategies to prevent in-hospital cardiac arrest: analysing responses of physicians and nurses in the hours before the event. *Critical Care Medicine* 1994; **22**: 244–247.
5. McQuillan P, Pilkington S, Allan A *et al.* Confidential enquiry into quality of care before admission to intensive care. *British Medical Journal* 1998; **316**: 1853–1858.
6. McGloin H, Adam SK and Singer M. Unexpected deaths and referrals to intensive care of patients on general wards: are some potentially avoidable? *Journal of the Royal College of Physicians* 1999; **33**: 255–259.
7. Goldhill DR and McNarry AF. Physiological abnormalities in early warning scores are related to mortality in adult inpatients. *British Journal of Anaesthesia* 2004; **92(6)**: 882–884.
8. Subbe CP, Kruger M, Rutherford P and Gemmel L. Validation of a modified early warning score in medical admissions. *Quarterly Journal of Medicine* 2001; **94**: 521–526.
9. Goldhill D. Medical emergency teams. *Care of the Critically Ill* 2000; **16(6)**: 209–212.
10. Pittard AJ. Out of our reach? Assessing the impact of introducing a critical care outreach service. *Anaesthesia* 2003; **58**: 874–910.
11. Buist MD, Moore GE, Bernard S, Waxman BP, Anderson JN and Nguyen TV. Effects of a medical emergency team on reduction of incidence of and mortality from unexpected cardiac arrests in hospital: a preliminary study. *British Medical Journal* 2002; **324**: 1–6.
12. Ball C, Kirkby M and Williams S. Effect of the critical care outreach team on patient survival to discharge from hospital and readmission to critical care: non-randomised population based study. *British Medical Journal* 2003; **327**: 1014–1017.
13. Bristow PJ, Hillman KM, Chey T *et al.* Rates of in-hospital arrests, deaths and intensive care admissions: the effect of a medical emergency team. *Medical Journal of Australia* 2000; **173**: 236–240.
14. Bellomo R, Goldsmith D, Uchino S *et al.* A prospective before-and-after trial of a medical emergency team. *Medical Journal of Australia* 2003; **179**: 283–287.
15. Safar P. Critical care medicine – quo vadis? *Critical Care Medicine* 1974; **2**: 1–5.
16. Audit Commission. *Critical to Success – The Place of Efficient and Effective Critical Care Services Within the Acute Hospital.* Audit Commission, London, October 1999.
17. Department of Health. *Comprehensive Critical Care – A Review of Adult Critical Care Services.* Department of Health, London, May 2000.

18. Lyons RA, Wareham K, Hutchings HA *et al*. Population requirement for adult critical care beds: a prospective quantitative and qualitative study. *Lancet* 2000; **355(9024)**: 595–598.

19. Royal College of Physicians of London. *Working Party Report On the Interface Between Acute General [Internal] Medicine and Critical Care*. Royal College of Physicians of London, London, May 2002.

20. MERIT study investigators. Introduction of the medical emergency team (MET) system: a cluster-randomised controlled trial. *Lancet* 2005; **365**: 2091–2097.

21. NCEPOD. An Acute Problem? A Report of the National Confidential Enquiry into Patient Outcome and Death. NCEPOD, London, 2005. www.ncepod.org.uk

22. Coni N and Webster S. Demography. *Lecture Notes on Geriatrics, 5th Edition*. Blackwell, London, 1998.

23. Vincent C, Neale G and Woloshynowych M. Adverse events in British hospitals: preliminary retrospective record review. *British Medical Journal* 2001; **322**: 517–519.

24. Cooper N, Forrest K and Cramp P. *Essential Guide to Generic Skills*. Blackwell Publishing, Oxford, 2006.

Further resources

- ALERT (Acute Life-threatening Events Recognition and Treatment) is a generic, multi-professional acute care course developed by the School of Postgraduate Medicine, University of Portsmouth, UK. http://web.port.ac.uk/alert/intro.htm
- IMPACT courses (Ill Medical Patients Acute Care and Treatment) are run by the Royal College of Physicians and Surgeons of Glasgow. www.rcpsglasg.ac.uk/education/pallevents.asp
- CCrISP courses (Care of the Critically Ill Surgical Patient) are run by the Royal College of Surgeons of England and Edinburgh. www.rcseng.ac.uk/courses (under basic surgical training)
- ALS (Advanced Life Support) and ILS (Intermediate Life Support) courses are run by the Resuscitation Council, UK. These centre on the management of cardiac arrest and peri-arrest scenarios. www.resus.org.uk
- ATLS courses (Advanced Trauma and Life Support) are run by the Royal College of Surgeons of England and Edinburgh and focus on trauma care. www.rcseng.ac.uk/courses (under basic surgical training)
- The National Patient Safety Agency (UK) – www.npsa.nhs.uk
- Contact your local Trust or Deanery (department for postgraduate medical education) for courses on teamwork and communication skills.

CHAPTER 2

Oxygen therapy

By the end of this chapter you will be able to:

- Prescribe oxygen therapy
- Understand the different devices used to deliver oxygen
- Understand the reasons why $PaCO_2$ rises
- Know the limitations of pulse oximetry
- Understand the principle of oxygen delivery
- Apply this to your clinical practice

Myths about oxygen

Oxygen was described by Joseph Priestley in 1777 and has become one of the most commonly used drugs in medical practice. Yet oxygen therapy is often described inaccurately, prescribed variably and understood little. In 2000 we carried out two surveys of oxygen therapy. The first looked at oxygen prescriptions for post-operative patients in a large district general hospital in the UK. It found that there were several dozen ways used to prescribe oxygen and that the prescriptions were rarely followed. The second asked 50 qualified medical and nursing staff working in acute areas about oxygen masks and the concentration of oxygen delivered by each [1]. They were also asked which mask was most appropriate for a range of clinical situations. The answers revealed that many staff could not name the different types of oxygen mask, the difference between oxygen flow and concentration was poorly understood, one third chose a 28% Venturi mask for an unwell asthmatic and very few staff understood that $PaCO_2$ rises most commonly due to reasons that have nothing to do with oxygen therapy.

Misunderstanding of oxygen therapy is widespread and the result is that many patients are treated suboptimally. Yet oxygen is a drug with a correct concentration and side effects.

Hypoxaemia and hypoxia

Hypoxaemia is defined as the reduction below normal levels of oxygen in arterial blood – a PaO_2 of less than 8.0 kPa (60 mmHg) or oxygen saturations less than 93%. The normal range for arterial blood oxygen is 11–14 kPa (85–105 mmHg) which reduces in old age. *Hypoxia* is the reduction below normal levels of oxygen in the tissues and leads to organ damage. Cyanosis is an unreliable indicator of hypoxaemia, since its presence also depends on the haemoglobin concentration.

The main causes of hypoxaemia are as follows:
- Hypoventilation
- Ventilation–perfusion (V/Q) mismatch
- Intrapulmonary shunt.

These are discussed further in Chapter 4. Tissue hypoxia can also be caused by circulation abnormalities and impaired oxygen utilisation, for example in severe sepsis (discussed further in Chapter 6).

Symptoms and signs of hypoxaemia include:
- Cyanosis
- Restlessness
- Palpitations
- Sweating
- Confusion
- Headache
- Hypertension then hypotension
- Reduced conscious level.

The goal of oxygen therapy is to correct alveolar and tissue hypoxia, aiming for a PaO_2 of at least 8.0 kPa (60 mmHg) or oxygen saturations of at least 93%. Aiming for oxygen saturations of 100% is usually unnecessary and wasteful.

Oxygen therapy

There are very few published guidelines on oxygen therapy for acutely ill patients. The American Association for Respiratory Care has published the following indications for oxygen therapy [2]:
- Hypoxaemia (PaO_2 less than 8.0 kPa/60 mmHg, or saturations less than 93%)
- An acute situation where hypoxaemia is suspected
- Severe trauma
- Acute myocardial infarction
- During surgery.

However, oxygen therapy is also indicated in the peri-operative period, for respiratory distress, shock, severe sepsis, carbon monoxide (CO) poisoning, severe anaemia and when drugs are used which reduce ventilation (e.g. opioids). Post-operative oxygen therapy reduces cardiac ischaemic events, and high-concentration oxygen therapy has been shown to reduce post-operative nausea and vomiting in certain patients and wound infections after colorectal surgery.

Oxygen masks are divided into two groups, depending on whether they deliver a proportion of, or the entire ventilatory requirement (Fig. 2.1):
1 *Low flow masks*: Nasal cannulae, Hudson (or MC) masks and reservoir bag masks.
2 *High flow masks*: Venturi masks.

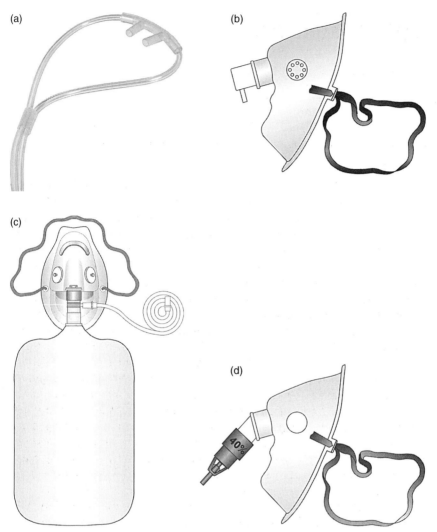

Figure 2.1 Different oxygen masks. (a) Nasal cannulae, (b) Hudson or MC mask, (c) Mask with a reservoir bag and (d) Venturi mask. Reproduced with permission from Intersurgical Complete Respiratory Systems, Wokingham, Berkshire.

Any oxygen delivery system can also be humidified. In common use in the UK is a humidified oxygen circuit which uses an adjustable Venturi valve.

Nasal cannulae
Nasal cannulae are commonly used because they are convenient and comfort-able. Nasal catheters (a single tube inserted into a nostril with a sponge) are also sometimes used. The oxygen flow rate does not usually exceed 4 l/min

Oxygen flow rate (l/min)	Inspired oxygen concentration (%)
1	24
2	28
3	32
4	36

Figure 2.2 Theoretical oxygen concentrations for nasal cannulae.

because this tends to be poorly tolerated by patients. If you look closely at the packaging of nasal cannulae, you will read that 2 l/min of oxygen via nasal cannulae delivers 28% oxygen. This statement makes many assumptions about the patient's pulmonary physiology. In fact, the concentration of oxygen delivered by nasal cannulae is variable both between patients and in the same patient at different times. The concentration is affected by factors such as the size of the anatomical reservoir and the peak inspiratory flow rate.

If you take a deep breath in, you will inhale approximately 1 l of air in a second. This is equivalent to an inspiratory flow rate of 60 l/min. The inspiratory flow rate varies throughout the respiratory cycle, hence there is also a *peak* inspiratory flow rate. Normal peak inspiratory flow rate is 40–60 l/min. But imagine for a moment that the inspiratory flow rate is constant. If a person has an inspiratory flow rate of 30 l/min and is given 2 l/min oxygen via nasal cannulae, he will inhale 2 l/min of pure oxygen and 28 l/min of air. If that same person changes his pattern of breathing so that the inspiratory flow rate rises to 60 l/min, the person will now inhale 2 l/min of pure oxygen and 58 l/min of air. In other words, a person with a higher inspiratory flow rate inhales proportionately less oxygen, and a person with a lower inspiratory flow rate inhales proportionately more oxygen. All low flow masks have this characteristic and therefore deliver a variable concentration of oxygen.

The *theoretical* oxygen concentrations for nasal cannulae at various flow rates are given in Fig. 2.2. These concentrations are a rough guide and apply to an average, healthy person. But because nasal cannulae in fact deliver a variable concentration of oxygen, there are several case reports on the 'dangers of low flow oxygen' during exacerbations of chronic obstructive pulmonary disease (COPD) [3] where low inspiratory flow rates can occur (and therefore higher oxygen concentrations).

Hudson or MC masks

Hudson or MC (named after Mary Catterall but also referred to as 'medium concentration') masks are also sometimes called 'simple face masks'. They are said to deliver around 50% oxygen when set to 10–15 l/min. The mask provides an additional 100–200 ml oxygen reservoir and that is why a higher concentration of oxygen is delivered compared with nasal cannulae. However, just like nasal cannulae, the concentration of oxygen delivered varies depending on the peak inspiratory flow rate as well as the fit of the mask. Importantly (and usually not known), significant rebreathing of CO_2 can occur if the oxygen flow rate is set to less than 5 l/min because exhaled air may not be adequately flushed from the mask. Nasal cannulae should be used if less than 5 l/min of low flow oxygen is required.

Reservoir bag masks

Reservoir bag masks are similar in design to Hudson masks, with the addition of a 600–1000-ml reservoir bag which increases the oxygen concentration still further. Reservoir bag masks are said to deliver around 80% oxygen at 10–15 l/min, but again this varies depending on the peak inspiratory flow rate as well as the fit of the mask. There are two types of reservoir bag mask: *partial rebreathe masks* and *non-rebreathe masks*. Partial rebreathe masks conserve oxygen supplies – useful if travelling with a cylinder. The first one-third of the patient's exhaled gas fills the reservoir bag, but as this is primarily from the anatomical deadspace, it contains little CO_2. The patient then inspires a mixture of exhaled gas and fresh gas (mainly oxygen). Non-rebreathe masks are so called because exhaled air exits the side of the mask through one-way valves and is prevented from entering the reservoir bag by another one-way valve. The patient therefore only inspires fresh gas (mainly oxygen). With both types of reservoir bag masks, the reservoir should be filled with oxygen before the mask is placed on the patient and the bag should not deflate by more than two-thirds with each breath in order to be effective. If the oxygen flow rate and oxygen reservoir are insufficient to meet the inspiratory demands of a patient with a particularly high inspiratory flow rate, the bag may collapse and the patient's oxygenation could be compromised. To prevent this, reservoir bag masks must be used with a minimum of 10 l/min of oxygen, and some are fitted with a spring-loaded tension valve which will open and allow entrainment of room air if necessary.

It is impossible for a patient to receive 100% oxygen via any mask for the simple reason that there is no airtight seal between mask and patient. Entrained air is always inspired as well.

Nasal cannulae, Hudson or MC masks, and reservoir bag masks all deliver a variable concentration of oxygen. They are all called low flow masks because the highest gas flow from the mask is 15 l/min, whereas a patient's inspiratory flow rate can be much higher. It is important to realise that low flow does not necessarily mean low concentration.

Venturi masks

Venturi masks, on the other hand, are high flow masks. The Venturi valve utilises the Bernoulli principle and has the effect of increasing the gas flow to above the patient's peak inspiratory flow rate (which is why these masks make more noise). A changing inspiratory pattern does not affect the oxygen concentration delivered, because the gas flow is high enough to meet the patient's peak inspiratory demands.

Bernoulli observed that fluid velocity increases at a constriction. This is what happens when you put your thumb over the end of a garden hose. If you were to look down a Venturi valve, you would observe a small hole. Oxygen is forced through this short constriction and the sudden subsequent increase in area creates a pressure gradient which increases velocity and entrains room air (see Fig. 2.3). At the patient's face there is a constant air–oxygen mixture which flows at a rate higher than the normal peak inspiratory flow rate. So changes in the pattern of breathing do not affect the oxygen concentration. There are two types of Venturi systems: colour-coded valve masks and a variable model. With colour-coded valve masks (labelled 24%, 28%, 35%, 40% and 60%), each is designed to deliver a fixed percentage of oxygen when set to the appropriate flow rate. To change the oxygen concentration, both the valve and flow have to be changed. The size of the orifice and the oxygen flow rate are different for each type of valve, because they have been calculated accordingly. The variable model is most commonly encountered in the UK with humidified oxygen circuits. The orifice is adjustable and the oxygen flow rate is set depending on what oxygen concentration is desired.

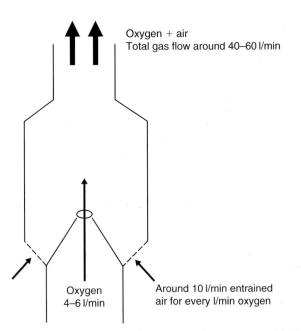

Oxygen + air
Total gas flow around 40–60 l/min

Oxygen
4–6 l/min

Around 10 l/min entrained
air for every l/min oxygen

Figure 2.3 A 28% Venturi mask. Bernoulli's equation for incompressible flow states that $1/2pv^2 + P$ = constant (where p is density) so if the pressure (P) of a gas falls, it gains velocity (v). When gas moves through the Venturi valve there is a sudden drop due to the increase in area. The velocity or flow of gas increases according to the above equation and entrains air as a result.

Venturi masks are the first choice in patients who require controlled oxygen therapy. The concentration of inspired oxygen is determined by the mask rather than the characteristics of the patient. Increasing the oxygen flow rate will increase total gas flow, but not the inspired oxygen concentration. However, with inspired oxygen concentrations of over 40%, the Venturi system may still not have enough total flow to meet high inspiratory demands. Fig. 2.4 shows the flow rates for various Venturi masks and Fig. 2.5 shows the effect of lower total flow rates in patients with high inspiratory demands.

Venturi valve colour	Inspired oxygen concentration (%)	Oxygen flow (l/min)	Total gas flow (l/min)
Blue	24	2–4	51–102
White	28	4–6	44–67
Yellow	35	8–10	45–65
Red	40	10–12	41–50
Green	60	12–15	24–30
Humidified circuit	85	12–15	15–20

Figure 2.4 Venturi mask flow rates. Data provided by Intersurgical Complete Respiratory Systems, Wokingham, Berkshire.

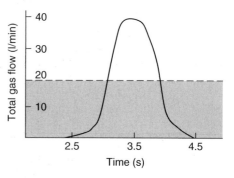

Figure 2.5 Lower total flow rates in patients with high inspiratory demands. Data provided by Intersurgical Complete Respiratory Systems, Wokingham, Berkshire.

- Venturi humidified oxygen circuit set to 85% with an oxygen flow rate of 15 l/min (total gas flow 20 l/min).

- The curve shows a patient's inspiratory flow pattern with a peak inspiratory flow rate of 40 l/min. The total gas flow is only 20 l/min, so for part of the inspiratory cycle, the patient is breathing mainly air. This reduces the overall inspired oxygen concentration to around 60%.

Humidified oxygen

Normally, inspired air is warmed and humidified to almost 90% by the nasopharynx. Administering dry oxygen lowers the water content of inspired air, even more so if an artificial airway bypasses the nasopharynx. This can result in ciliary dysfunction, impaired mucous transport, retention of secretions, atelectasis, and even bacterial infiltration of the pulmonary mucosa and pneumonia. Humidified oxygen is given to avoid this, and is particularly important when prolonged high-concentration oxygen is administered and in pneumonia or post-operative respiratory failure where the expectoration of secretions is important.

In summary, flow is not the same as concentration! Low flow masks can deliver high concentrations of oxygen and high flow masks can deliver low concentrations of oxygen. Therefore, the terms 'high concentration' and 'low concentration' should be used when discussing oxygen therapy. Furthermore, when giving instructions or prescribing oxygen therapy, two parts are required: the type of mask *and* the flow rate. You cannot simply say '28%' as this is meaningless – one person might assume this means a 28% Venturi mask, and another may assume this means 2 l/min via nasal cannulae. If the patient has an exacerbation of COPD, this difference could be important.

Why are there so many different types of oxygen mask? Nasal cannulae are convenient and comfortable. Patients can easily speak, eat and drink wearing nasal cannulae. Reservoir bag masks deliver the highest concentrations of oxygen and should always be available in acute areas. A fixed concentration of oxygen is important for many patients, as is humidified oxygen. Since Venturi masks deliver a range of oxygen concentrations from 24% to 60%, some hospital departments in the UK choose not to stock Hudson (MC) masks as well. Fig. 2.6 shows which mask is appropriate for different clinical situations and Fig. 2.7 shows a simple guide to oxygen therapy. Oxygen therapy should be goal directed. The right patient should receive the right amount of oxygen for the right length of time.

Oxygen mask	Clinical situation
Nasal cannulae (2–4 l/min)	Patients with otherwise normal vital signs (e.g. post-operative, slightly low SpO_2, long-term oxygen therapy).
Hudson masks (more than 5 l/min) or reservoir bag masks (more than 10 l/min)	Higher concentrations required and controlled oxygen not necessary (e.g. severe asthma, acute left ventricular failure, pneumonia, trauma, severe sepsis).
Venturi masks	Controlled oxygen therapy required (e.g. patients with exacerbation of COPD).

Figure 2.6 Which mask for which patient?

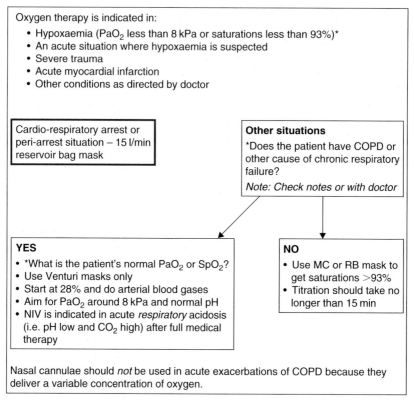

Figure 2.7 A simple guide to oxygen therapy.

Can oxygen therapy be harmful?

Hyperoxaemia can sometimes have adverse effects. Prolonged exposure to high concentrations of oxygen (above 50%) can lead to atelectasis and acute lung injury, usually in an ICU setting. Absorption atelectasis occurs as nitrogen is washed out of the alveoli and oxygen is readily absorbed into the bloodstream, leaving the alveoli to collapse. Acute lung injury is thought to be due to oxygen free radicals. Hyperoxaemia can increase systemic vascular resistance which may be a disadvantage in some patients. Oxygen is also combustible. There is also a group of patients with chronic respiratory failure who may develop hypercapnia when given high concentrations of oxygen, a fact which is usually emphasised in undergraduate medical teaching.

But!!!

Hypoxaemia kills. There have been cases of negligence in which doctors have withheld oxygen therapy from acutely ill patients due to an unfounded fear of exacerbating hypercapnia. The next section will discuss in detail the causes of hypercapnia with special reference to oxygen therapy, and the role of acute oxygen therapy in patients with chronic respiratory failure, particularly COPD.

Hypercapnia and oxygen therapy

From a physiological point of view, $PaCO_2$ rises for the following reasons:

- Alveolar hypoventilation (alveolar ventilation is the portion of ventilation which takes part in gas exchange; it is not the same as a reduced respiratory rate).
- V/Q mismatch. PaO_2 falls and $PaCO_2$ rises when blood flow is increased to poorly ventilated areas of lung and the patient cannot compensate by an overall increase in alveolar ventilation.
- Increased CO_2 production (e.g. severe sepsis, malignant hyperthermia, bicarbonate infusion) where the patient cannot compensate by an overall increase in alveolar ventilation.
- Increased inspired $PaCO_2$ (e.g. breathing into a paper bag).

Fig. 2.8 shows how respiratory muscle load and respiratory muscle strength can become affected by disease and an imbalance leads to alveolar hypoventilation and hypercapnia. Respiratory muscle load is increased by increased resistance (e.g. upper or lower airway obstruction), reduced compliance (e.g. infection, oedema, rib fractures or obesity) and increased respiratory rate. Respiratory muscle strength can be reduced by a problem in any part of the neurorespiratory pathway: motor neurone disease, Guillain–Barré syndrome, myasthenia gravis or electrolyte abnormalities (low potassium, magnesium, phosphate or calcium). It is important to realise that alveolar hypoventilation usually occurs with a high (but ineffective) respiratory rate, as opposed to total hypoventilation (a reduced respiratory rate) which is usually caused by drug overdose.

A problem with ventilation is the most common cause of hypercapnia among hospital in-patients. Examples include the overdose patient with airway obstruction, the 'tired' asthmatic, the morbidly obese patient with pneumonia, the patient with post-operative respiratory failure on an opioid infusion, the trauma patient with rib fractures and pulmonary contusions, the pancreatitis patient with acute respiratory distress syndrome, the patient with acute pulmonary oedema on the coronary care unit and so on.

In other words, oxygen therapy is an uncommon cause of hypercapnia.

There are many conditions in which chronic hypercapnia occurs: severe chest wall deformity, morbid obesity and neurological conditions causing

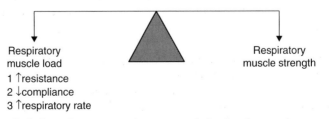

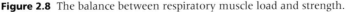

Figure 2.8 The balance between respiratory muscle load and strength.

muscle weakness, for example. The reasons for chronic hypercapnia in COPD are not really known, but are thought to include a low chemical drive for breathing, genetic factors and an acquired loss of drive due to adaptation to increased work of breathing. Chronic hypercapnia in COPD tends to occur when the forced expiratory volume (FEV_1) is less than 1 l.

For the purposes of explanation here, the term 'CO_2 retention' will be used to describe acute hypercapnia when patients with chronic respiratory failure are given high-concentration (or uncontrolled) oxygen therapy. 'Ventilatory failure' will be used to describe acute hypercapnia due to other causes.

CO_2 retention

In 1949 a case was described of a man with emphysema who lapsed into a coma after receiving oxygen therapy but rapidly recovered after the oxygen was removed [4]. In 1954 a decrease in ventilation was observed in 26 out of 35 patients with COPD given oxygen therapy, with a rise in $PaCO_2$ and a fall in pH. No patient with a normal baseline PaO_2 showed these changes [5]. In a further study it was showed that stopping and starting oxygen therapy led to a fall and rise in $PaCO_2$, respectively [6]. These early experiments led to the concept of 'hypoxic drive', proposed by Campbell [7], which is taught in medical schools today. The teaching goes like this: changes in $PaCO_2$ is one of the main controls of ventilation in normal people. In patients with a chronically high $PaCO_2$ the chemoreceptors in the brain become blunted and the patient depends on hypoxaemia to stimulate ventilation, something which normally occurs only at altitude or during illness. If these patients are given too much oxygen, their 'hypoxic drive' is abolished, breathing will slow and $PaCO_2$ will rise as a result, causing CO_2 narcosis and eventually apnoea.

Unfortunately, hypoxic drive is not responsible for the rise in $PaCO_2$ seen when patients with chronic respiratory failure are given uncontrolled oxygen therapy. Subsequent studies have questioned this theory and it is now thought that changes in V/Q are more important in the aetiology of CO_2 retention. Hypoxic vasoconstriction is a normal physiological mechanism in the lungs. When oxygen therapy is given to patients with chronic hypoxemia, this is reversed leading to changes in V/Q. $PaCO_2$ rises because more CO_2-containing blood is delivered to less well-ventilated areas of lung. In a person with a normal chemical drive for breathing, this would be compensated for by an overall increase in alveolar ventilation. But if the chemical drive for breathing is impaired (as in some patients with COPD), or there are mechanical limitations to increasing ventilation, or fatigue, this cannot occur. In other words, the combination of changes in V/Q plus the inability to compensate is why CO_2 retention occurs. Studies have failed to show a reduction in minute ventilation to account for this phenomenon, although it is possible it may contribute in some way [8,9].

Which patients are at risk of CO_2 retention? The answer is patients with chronic respiratory failure. It is not the label 'COPD', but the presence of chronic respiratory failure, which occurs in other diseases as well, that is important. Some patients with COPD are fairly physiologically normal. This may explain the studies which show no significant change in $PaCO_2$ when patients with an exacerbation of COPD were given high-concentration oxygen therapy. In one study, patients with a PaO_2 of less than 6.6 kPa (50 mmHg) and a $PaCO_2$ of more than 6.6 kPa (50 mmHg) were randomised to receive oxygen therapy either to get the PaO_2 just above 6.6 kPa or above 9 kPa (70 mmHg). There was no significant difference between the two groups in terms of mortality, need for ventilation, duration of hospital stay, $PaCO_2$ or pH despite a significant difference in PaO_2. There was a trend towards improved outcome in the higher oxygen group [10].

Half of admissions with an acute exacerbation of COPD have reversible hypercapnia [11,12]. In other words, these people have acute but not chronic respiratory failure. Non-invasive ventilation has been shown to be a very successful treatment for acute respiratory failure (or acute on chronic respiratory failure) in COPD, leading to a reduction in mortality and length of hospital stay [13]. How can you tell if a patient with COPD has a high $PaCO_2$ because of oxygen therapy (CO_2 retention) or because they are sick (ventilatory failure), and does it matter, since the treatment is essentially the same: controlled oxygen therapy titrated to arterial blood gases, medical therapy and ventilation if needed?

Fig. 2.9 is a simplified guide to the clinical differences between CO_2 retainers and patients with ventilatory failure and COPD. Of course, many patients

Likely CO_2 retention	Likely ventilatory failure
Usually severely limited by breathlessness	Not usually limited by breathlessness
Cor pulmonale or polycythaemia present	No signs of chronic hypoxaemia
FEV_1 less than 1 l	FEV_1 good
On home nebulisers and/or home oxygen	Inhalers only
Abnormal blood gases when well	Normal blood gases when well
Admission blood gases show pH and st bicarbonate/BE consistent with chronic hypercapnia	Admission blood gases show pH and st bicarbonate/BE consistent with critical illness
Vital signs and oxygen saturations not very different to normal	Critically ill
Reasonable air entry	Silent chest or feeble chest movements
	Dubious diagnosis of COPD
	Chest X-ray shows pulmonary oedema or severe pneumonia

Figure 2.9 CO_2 retention due to oxygen therapy vs ventilatory failure in patients with COPD.

will fall in between these two extremes (in which case a pragmatic approach is required), but it is nevertheless a useful guide, especially when teaching.

One in five patients with COPD admitted to hospital has a respiratory acidosis. The more severe the acidosis, the greater the mortality. Some of these acidoses may be caused by uncontrolled oxygen therapy, since a proportion disappears quickly after arrival in hospital [14], although this may also be due to treatment with bronchodilators. Recent UK National Institute for Clinical Excellence (NICE) guidelines recommend using Venturi masks in conjunction with pulse oximetry for exacerbations of COPD, increasing or reducing the oxygen to maintain saturations of 90–93%, until further information can be gained from arterial blood gases [15]. Despite such guidelines, oxygen therapy in COPD continues to cause controversy. This may be because patients with COPD constitute a physiologically diverse group and so there can be no 'rules'. For example, in 2002, the journal *Clinical Medicine* published an audit of oxygen therapy in acute exacerbations of COPD [16]. One hundred and one admissions were analysed and 57% of patients received more than 28% oxygen on their way to hospital. The median duration from ambulance to first arterial blood gas was 1 h. Half of the patients identified their illness incorrectly as 'asthma' to the ambulance crew. Controversially, the audit found that in-hospital mortality was greater in those patients who received more than 28% oxygen and postulated that there was a causal relationship. The publication of this article was followed by the publication of a strongly worded letter by two eminent critical care physicians and it is worth reading in full [17]. They strongly disagreed with the assumptions behind the article, and among other things, pointed out that nearly all studies involving patients with an acute exacerbation of COPD ignore the base deficit in their comparisons of outcome and mention only pH, $PaCO_2$ and PaO_2. Since the base deficit is known to correlate strongly with mortality [18], outcome studies which ignore it are meaningless. They finished by saying, 'we frequently attend A&E departments to treat [patients with an exacerbation of COPD] and routinely use high-concentration oxygen, despite a high $PaCO_2$, in conjunction with mechanical ventilation (invasive or non-invasive) because their major problem is fatigue, often compounded by atelectasis due to shallow respiratory efforts, weak cough and sputum retention, rather than the semi-mythical loss of hypoxic drive. To allow them to remain hypoxaemic (i.e. below their normal baseline) and thus struggle and tire further is contrary to all the precepts underpinning ABC resuscitation and good clinical practice. Remarkably, our patients often do very well. As a simple rule of thumb, hypoxic drive is a non-issue in tachypnoeic patients'.

The answer to the question 'How much oxygen should be given in an exacerbation of COPD?' is therefore: enough, monitored closely and in conjunction with other treatments.

To summarise:

- The most common cause of hypercapnia for hospital in-patients is acute illness causing ventilatory failure. This has nothing to do with oxygen therapy – treat the cause.

- In patients with chronic respiratory failure, start with a 28% Venturi mask and titrate oxygen therapy to arterial blood gases (see Fig. 2.7).
- Controlled oxygen therapy, medical treatment and mechanical ventilation are used to treat acute respiratory acidosis (low pH due to a high $PaCO_2$) in an exacerbation of COPD.

Pulse oximetry

Oximetry works on the principle that light is absorbed by a solution, and the degree of absorption is related to the molar concentration of that solution (Fig. 2.10). The Lambert and Beer laws describe this. Oxyhaemoglobin (HbO_2) and de-oxyhaemoglobin (Hb) have different absorbencies at certain wavelengths of light (660 and 940 nm). There are two ways to measure haemoglobin oxygen saturation using oximetry: by a *co-oximeter* or a *pulse oximeter*. A co-oximeter haemolyses blood and is a component of most blood gas machines. It measures SaO_2. A pulse oximeter consists of a peripheral probe and a central processing and

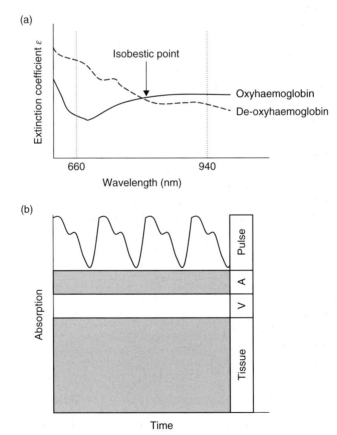

Figure 2.10 (a) Absorption in a pulse oximeter and (b) components of absorption: tissue, venous blood (V), arterial blood (A) and pulsatile arterial blood.

display unit. It measures SpO$_2$. Two light emitting diodes (LEDs) in the probe of a pulse oximeter transilluminate separate pulses of light in the red and infrared spectra, and the absorbance is measured by a photodiode on the other side, enabling the concentration of HbO$_2$ and Hb, and therefore haemoglobin saturation to be calculated. This is the 'functional saturation' as further calculations are then done to account for minor haemoglobin species. The probe is able to correct for ambient light. As blood flow is pulsatile, the transilluminated signal consists of an 'AC' component as well as a 'DC' component (which represents the light absorbed by tissues and resting blood). Although the AC component is a small proportion of the total signal, it is a major determinant of accuracy, which explains why pulse oximeters are inaccurate in low perfusion states.

Oximeters are calibrated by the manufacturers using data that was originally obtained by human volunteers. SpO$_2$ was measured while the volunteers inspired various oxygen concentrations. Due to this, they are only accurate between 80% and 100% saturation, as it was unethical to calibrate oximeters below this point.

Oxygen saturation *indirectly* relates to arterial oxygen content (PaO$_2$) through the oxygen dissociation curve. Remembering this indirect relationship is

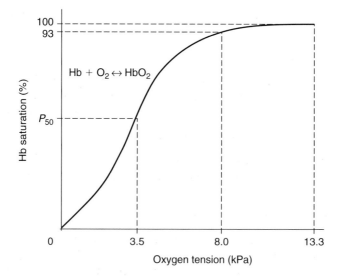

- The oxygen dissociation curve falls sharply after saturation of 93% (8.0 kPa). SpO$_2$ of 93% or less is abnormal and requires assessment.
- The curve is shifted to the right in fever, raised 2,3-diphosphoglycerate (2,3-DPG) and acidosis (the shift caused by pH is called the Bohr effect). This means P_{50} increases and higher pulmonary capillary saturations are required to saturate Hb, but there is enhanced delivery at the tissues.
- The curve is shifted to the left by hypothermia, reduced 2,3-DPG, alkalosis and the presence of foetal Hb. This means P_{50} reduces and lower pulmonary capillary saturations are required to saturate Hb, but lower tissue capillary PaO$_2$ is required before oxygen is delivered.

Figure 2.11 The oxygen dissociation curve.

important, because SpO_2 is affected by several internal factors (see Fig. 2.11) as well as external factors, listed below. It is also important to remember that SpO_2 is only a measure of oxygenation, not ventilation.

The technical limitations of pulse oximetry include the following:

- Motion artefact – excessive movement (e.g. in the back of an ambulance) interferes with the signal.
- External light from fluorescent lighting and poorly shielded probes also interferes with the signal.
- An ill-fitting probe may give spurious readings.
- Injectable dyes such as methylene blue can interfere with SpO_2 readings for several hours.
- Dark nail polish may interfere with the signal.
- Anaemia – at a Hb of 8 g/dl the oxygen saturation is underestimated by 10–15%, especially at lower saturation levels.
- Vasoconstriction and poor tissue perfusion give low amplitude signals which increase error. Modern oximeters display 'poor signal' messages.
- Abnormal haemoglobins – methaemoglobin reduces SpO_2 despite a normal PaO_2, and carboxyhaemoglobin is not detected by pulse oximetry despite a low PaO_2.

Dark skin has been studied and does not affect the accuracy of pulse oximetry.

Oxygen delivery

Tissues need oxygen to metabolise. Nearly all oxygen is carried to the tissues by haemoglobin. Each g/dl of haemoglobin carries 1.3 ml of oxygen when fully saturated. The oxygen content of blood can therefore be calculated as:

Hb (g/dl) $\times$ oxygen saturation of Hb $\times$ 1.3

Haemoglobin is delivered to the tissues by the circulation. The amount of oxygen delivered per minute depends on the cardiac output. From this we derive the oxygen delivery equation:

Hb($\times$10 to convert to litres) $\times$ SaO_2 $\times$ 1.3 $\times$ CO(l/min)

Oxygen delivery is an important concept in intensive care medicine. In fact, the importance of oxygen delivery explains the emphasis on airway, breathing and circulation (ABC) in teaching acute care. Understanding that oxygen *delivery* depends on more than just oxygen *therapy* will help you optimise your patient's condition. In the ICU, oxygen delivery is manipulated in high-tech ways. The following is a simple ward-based example: in a 70-kg man a normal Hb is 14 g/dl, normal SaO_2 is 95% and normal cardiac output is 5 l/min. Oxygen delivery is therefore $14 \times 0.95 \times 1.3 \times 10 \times 5 = 864.5$ ml O_2/min. Imagine this patient now has severe pneumonia and is dehydrated. His SaO_2 is 93% and he has a reduced cardiac output (4 l/min). His oxygen delivery is $14 \times 0.93 \times 1.3 \times 10 \times 4 = 677$ ml O_2/min. By increasing his oxygen so that his saturations are now 98% his oxygen delivery can be increased to

713 ml O_2/min, but if a fluid challenge is given to increase his cardiac output to normal (5 l/min), yet his oxygen is kept the same, his oxygen delivery can be increased to 846 ml O_2/min. Oxygen delivery has been increased more by giving fluid than by giving oxygen.

The oxygen delivery equation also illustrates the relationship between SaO_2 and haemoglobin. An SaO_2 of 95% with severe anaemia is worse in terms of oxygen delivery than an SaO_2 of 80% with a haemoglobin of 15 g/dl, and this is why patients with chronic hypoxaemia develop polycythaemia.

Key points: oxygen therapy

- The goal of oxygen therapy is to correct alveolar and tissue hypoxia, aiming for a PaO_2 of at least 8.0 kPa (60 mmHg) or oxygen saturations of at least 93%.
- Oxygen masks are divided into two groups: *low flow masks* which deliver a variable concentration of oxygen (nasal cannulae, Hudson or MC masks and reservoir bag masks) and *high flow Venturi masks* which deliver a fixed concentration of oxygen.
- The most common cause of hypercapnia for hospital in-patients is ventilatory failure. This has nothing to do with oxygen therapy – treat the cause.
- Pulse oximetry is a measure of oxygenation, not ventilation.

Self-assessment: case histories

1 A 60-year-old woman arrives in the Emergency Department with breathlessness. She was given 12 l/min oxygen via simple face mask by the paramedics. She is on inhalers for COPD, is a smoker and has diabetes. She is clammy and has widespread crackles and wheeze in the lungs. The chest X-ray has an appearance consistent with severe left ventricular failure. Her blood gases are: pH 7.15, $PaCO_2$ 8.0 kPa (61.5 mmHg), PaO_2 9.0 kPa (69.2 mmHg), st bicarbonate 20 mmol/l, base excess (BE) −6. The attending doctor has taken the oxygen mask off because of 'CO$_2$ retention' by the time you arrive. The oxygen saturations were 95% and are now 85%. Blood pressure is 180/70 mmHg. Comment on her oxygen therapy. What is your management?

2 A 50-year-old man arrives in the Medical Admissions Unit with breathlessness. He is an ex-miner, has COPD and is on inhalers at home. His blood gases on 28% oxygen show: pH 7.4, $PaCO_2$ 8.5 kPa (65.3 mmHg), PaO_2 8.5 kPa (65.3 mmHg), st bicarbonate 38.4 mmol/l, BE +7. A colleague asks you if he needs non-invasive ventilation because of his hypercapnia. What is your reply?

3 A 40-year-old patient on the chemotherapy ward becomes unwell with breathlessness. The nurses report oxygen saturations of 75%. When you go to the patient, you find the other observations are as follows: pulse

130/min, blood pressure 70/40 mmHg, respiratory rate 40/min, patient confused. Blood gases on air show: pH 7.1, $PaCO_2$ 3.0 kPa (23 mmHg), PaO_2 13 kPa (115 mmHg), st bicarbonate 6.8 mmol/l, BE −20. The chest is clear. A chest X-ray is taken and is normal. Can you explain the oxygen saturations and the breathlessness? What is your management?

4 A 50-year-old man is undergoing a urological procedure. As part of this, intravenous methylene blue is given. Shortly afterwards, the junior anaesthetist notices the patient's oxygen saturations drop suddenly to 70%. All the equipment seems to be working normally. Worried that the patient has had some kind of embolism, he calls his senior. What is the explanation?

5 A 45-year-old man arrives unconscious in the Emergency Department. There is no history available apart from he was found collapsed in his car by passers-by. On examination he is unresponsive, pulse 90/min, blood pressure 130/60 mmHg, oxygen saturations 98% on 15 l/min oxygen via reservoir bag mask. His ECG shows widespread ST depression and his arterial blood gases show: pH 7.25, $PaCO_2$ 6.0 kPa (46 mmHg), PaO_2 7.5 kPa (57.6 mmHg), st bicarbonate 19.4 mmol/l, BE −10. His full blood count is normal. What is the explanation for the discrepancy in the SpO_2 and PaO_2? What is your management?

6 A 25-year-old man with no past medical history was found on the floor at home having taken a mixed overdose of benzodiazepines and tricyclic antidepressant tablets. He responds only to painful stimuli (Glasgow Coma Score of 8) and he has probably aspirated, because there is right upper lobe consolidation on his chest X-ray. He is hypothermic (34°C) and arterial blood gases on 15 l/min via reservoir bag mask show: pH 7.2, $PaCO_2$ 9.5 kPa (73 mmHg), PaO_2 12.0 kPa (92.3 mmHg), st bicarbonate 27.3 mmol/l, BE −2. His blood pressure is 80/50 mmHg and his pulse is 120/min. The attending doctor changes his oxygen to a 28% Venturi mask because of his high CO_2 and repeat blood gases show: pH 7.2, $PaCO_2$ 9.0 kPa (69.2 mmHg), PaO_2 6.0 kPa (46.1 mmHg), st bicarbonate 26 mmol/l, BE −2. What would your management be?

7 A 70-year-old woman with severe COPD (FEV_1 0.6) is admitted with a chest infection and breathlessness far worse than usual. She is agitated on arrival and refuses to wear an oxygen mask. She is therefore given 2 l/min oxygen via nasal cannulae. Half-an-hour later, when the doctor arrives to re-assess her, she is unresponsive. What do you think has happened?

8 A 50-year-old man is recovering from an exacerbation of COPD in hospital. When you go to review him on the ward, you notice that he is being given 2 l/min of oxygen via a Hudson mask. Is this appropriate?

Self-assessment: discussion

1 The fact that this patient is 'on inhalers for COPD' does not mean that she actually has a diagnosis of COPD. How was this diagnosis made – on the basis of some breathlessness on exertion and her smoking history, or by

spirometry (the recommended standard)? Even if the diagnosis of COPD is established, is it mild or severe? Her current problem is not COPD at all, but acute severe cardiogenic pulmonary oedema, a condition which causes ventilatory failure. In a 60-year-old smoker with diabetes, a myocardial infarction is a likely cause. Acute hypoxaemia will aggravate cardiac ischaemia and this needs to be borne in mind. The arterial blood gases show a mixed respiratory and metabolic acidosis with relative hypoxaemia. Rather than removing the oxygen in the vague hope that this will 'treat' her high CO_2 (which it will not), this patient requires adequate oxygen therapy and treatment for acute left ventricular failure. If optimal medical therapy fails to improve things (i.v. furosemide and nitrates, nebulised salbutamol, with i.v. diamorphine in some patients), non-invasive continuous positive airway pressure (CPAP) may be tried before tracheal intubation and ventilation.

2 No. His pH is normal. Non-invasive ventilation is used for an exacerbation of COPD when the pH falls below normal due to a high $PaCO_2$. This patient has a high st bicarbonate, presumably in compensation for his chronically high $PaCO_2$. He should stay on a Venturi mask while unwell.

3 The main reason why this patient's oxygen saturations are so low is poor perfusion. The PaO_2 is normal on air – this makes pulmonary embolism unlikely in someone so unwell (cancer and chemotherapy are two independent risk factors for pulmonary embolism). This patient is in shock (circulatory failure) as illustrated by the low blood pressure and severe metabolic acidosis on the arterial blood gases. Shocked patients breathe faster because of tissue hypoxia as well as metabolic acidosis. The history and examination will tell you whether or not this shock is due to bleeding (Are the platelets very low?) or severe sepsis (Is the white cell count very low?). Patients with septic shock do not always have the classical warm peripheries and bounding pulses – they can be peripherally vasoconstricted. Management starts with A (airway with oxygen), B (breathing) and C (circulation) (see Box 1.3). This patient requires fluid and you should call for senior help immediately.

4 Methylene blue in the circulation affects the oxygen saturation measurement. Nevertheless, a concerned junior anaesthetist would check the airway (tube position), breathing (listen to the chest and check the ventilator settings) and circulation (measure blood pressure, pulse and assess perfusion) as well as asking for advice.

5 The arterial blood gases show a metabolic acidosis with hypoxaemia. The $PaCO_2$ is at the upper limit of normal. It should be low in a metabolic acidosis, indicating a relative respiratory acidosis as well. Treatment priorities in this patient are as follows: securing the airway and administering high-concentration oxygen, assessing and treating breathing, and correcting any circulation problems. There is a discrepancy between the SpO_2 of 98% and the arterial blood gas result which shows a PaO_2 of 7.5 kPa (57.6 mmHg). Tied in with the history and ischaemic-looking ECG, the explanation for this is carbon monoxide (CO) poisoning. CO poisoning produces COHb which is

Oxygen concentration	Half-life of CO (min)
Room air (21%)	240–300
15 l/min reservoir bag mask (80%)	80–100
Intubated and ventilated with 100% oxygen	50–70
Hyperbaric chamber (100% oxygen at 3 atm)	20–25

Figure 2.12 Half-life of CO depending on conditions.

interpreted by pulse oximeters as HbO_2 causing an overestimation of oxygen saturation. CO poisoning a common cause of death by poisoning in the UK. Mortality is especially high in those with pre-existing atherosclerosis. CO binds strongly to haemoglobin and causes the oxygen dissociation curve to shift to the left, leading to impaired oxygen transport and utilisation. Loss of CO from the body is a slow process at normal atmospheric pressure and oxygen concentration (21%). It takes 4.5 h for the concentration of CO to fall to half its original value. CO removal is increased by increasing the oxygen concentration or by placing the victim in a hyperbaric chamber. This increases the amount of oxygen in the blood, forcing off CO (see Fig. 2.12). Blood gas analysers use co-oximeters which can differentiate between COHb and HbO_2.

There is debate as to whether treatment with hyperbaric oxygen is superior to ventilation with 100% oxygen on an ICU. Five randomised trials to date disagree. Therefore a pragmatic approach is recommended. The following are features which should lead to consideration of hyperbaric oxygen therapy:
- Any history of unconsciousness
- COHb levels of greater than 40% at any time
- Neurological or psychiatric features at the time of examination
- Pregnancy (because the foetal COHb curve is shifted to the left of the mother's)
- ECG changes.

The risks of transporting critically ill patients to a hyperbaric unit also need to be taken into account. Ventilation with 100% oxygen is an acceptable alternative and this treatment should continue for a minimum of 12 h.

6 This is a 25-year-old man with no previous medical problems. He does not have chronic respiratory failure. He will not 'retain CO_2' – he has a problem with ventilation. The arterial blood gases show an acute respiratory acidosis with a lower PaO_2 than expected. He requires tracheal intubation to protect his airway and high-concentration oxygen (15 l/min via reservoir bag mask). He has several reasons to have a problem with ventilation – a reduced conscious level and possible airway obstruction, aspiration pneumonia and the respiratory depressant effects of his overdose. His hypotension should be treated with warmed fluid challenges. The drugs he has

taken (which cause cardiac toxicity) combined with hypoxaemia and hypoperfusion could lead to cardiac arrest. Intravenous sodium bicarbonate is indicated in severe tricyclic poisoning. Flumazenil (a benzodiazepine antidote) is not advised when significant amounts of tricyclic antidepressants have also been taken as this will reduce the seizure threshold. It is worth measuring creatinine kinase levels in this case as rhabdomyolysis (from lying on the floor for a long time due to drug overdose) would significantly affect fluid management.

7 This case illustrates the fact that 2 l/min via nasal cannulae is not the same as 28% oxygen via a Venturi mask, despite the theoretical oxygen concentrations displayed on the packaging of nasal cannulae. This lady is unconscious because of a high $PaCO_2$. This has happened either because her clinical condition deteriorated anyway, or because she has (inadvertently) been given a higher concentration of oxygen, or both. As always, start with A (airway), B (breathing – does she need ventilation?), C (circulation) and D (disability) before blood gas analysis.

8 This is a common scenario. Hudson or MC masks must always be set to a minimum of 5 l/min. Significant rebreathing of CO_2 can occur if the oxygen flow rate is set to less than this, because exhaled air may not be adequately flushed from the mask. The way to give low flow oxygen therapy at 2 l/min is to use nasal cannulae.

References

1. Cooper NA. Oxygen therapy – myths and misconceptions. *Care of the Critically Ill* 2002; **18(3)**: 74–77.
2. Kallstrom TJ. AARC clinical practice guideline. Oxygen therapy for adults in the acute care facility. *Respiratory Care* 2002; **47(6)**: 717–720.
3. Davies RJO and Hopkin JM. Nasal oxygen in exacerbations of ventilatory failure: an underappreciated risk. *British Medical Journal* 1989; **299**: 43–44.
4. Donald KW. Neurological effect of oxygen. *Lancet* 1949; **ii**: 1056–1057.
5. Prime FJ and Westlake EK. The respiratory response to CO_2 in emphysema. *Clinical Science* 1954; **13**: 321–332.
6. Westlake EK, Simpson T and Kaye M. Carbon dioxide narcosis in emphysema. *Quarterly Journal of Medicine* 1955; **94**: 155–173.
7. Campbell EJM. The management of respiratory failure in chronic bronchitis and emphysema. *American Review of Respiratory Disease* 1967; **96**: 626–639.
8. Aubier M, Murciano D, Milic-Emili J *et al*. Effects of administration of oxygen on ventilation and blood gases in patients with chronic obstructive pulmonary disease. *American Review of Respiratory Disease* 1980; **122**: 191–199.
9. Hanson III CW, Marshal BE, Frasch HF *et al*. Causes of hypercarbia with oxygen therapy in patients with chronic obstructive pulmonary disease. *Critical Care Medicine* 1996; **24**: 23–28.
10. Gomersal CD, Joynt GM, Freebairn RC, Lai CKW and Oh TE. Oxygen therapy for hypercapnic patients with chronic obstructive pulmonary disease and acute respiratory failure: a randomised controlled pilot study. *Critical Care Medicine* 2002; **30(1)**: 113–116.

11. Costello R, Deegan P, Fitzpatrick M *et al*. Reversible hypercapnia in chronic obstructive pulmonary disease: a distinct pattern of respiratory failure with a favourable prognosis. *American Journal of Medicine* 1997; **102**: 239–244.

12. McNally E, Fitzpatrick M and Bourke S. Reversible hypercapnia in acute exacerbations of chronic obstructive pulmonary disease (COPD). *European Respiratory Journal* 1993; **6**: 1353–1356.

13. Plant PK, Owen JL and Elliot MW. The YONIV trial. A multi-centre randomised controlled trial of the use of early non-invasive ventilation for exacerbations of chronic obstructive pulmonary disease on general respiratory wards. *Lancet* 2000; **355**: 1931–1935.

14. Plant PK, Owen JL and Elliot MW. One year period prevalence study of respiratory acidosis in acute exacerbations of COPD: implications for the provision of non-invasive ventilation and oxygen administration. *Thorax* 2000; **55**: 550–554.

15. British Thoracic Society. Guidelines for the management of acute exacerbations of COPD. *Thorax* 1997; **52(Suppl 5)**: S16–S21.

16. Denniston AKO, O'Brien C and Stableforth D. The use of oxygen in acute exacerbations of chronic obstructive pulmonary disease: a prospective audit of pre-hospital and emergency management. *Clinical Medicine* 2002; **2(5)**: 449–451.

17. Singer M and Bellingan G. Letter to the Editor. *Clinical Medicine* 2003; **3(2)**: 184.

18. Smith I, Kumar P, Molloy S, Rhodes A *et al*. Base excess and lactate as prognostic indicators for patients admitted to intensive care. *Intensive Care Medicine* 2001; **27**: 74–83.

Further resources

- www.brit-thoracic.org.uk/iqs/bts_guidelines_copd_html (COPD guidelines with link to the National Institute for Clinical Excellence guidelines)
- Moyle, J. *Pulse Oximetry*. BMJ Books, London, 2002.

CHAPTER 3

Acid–base balance

> **By the end of this chapter you will be able to:**
> - Understand how the body maintains a narrow pH
> - Know the meaning of common terms used in arterial blood gas analysis
> - Know the causes of acid–base abnormalities
> - Use a simple system to interpret arterial blood gases
> - Understand why arterial blood gases are an important test in critical illness
> - Apply this to your clinical practice

Acid as a by-product of metabolism

The human body is continually producing acid as a by-product of metabolism. But it must also maintain a narrow pH range, necessary for normal enzyme activity and the millions of chemical reactions that take place in the body each day. Normal blood pH is 7.35–7.45 and this is maintained by:
- Intracellular buffers (e.g. proteins and phosphate)
- Extracellular buffers (e.g. plasma proteins, haemoglobin and carbonic acid/bicarbonate)
- Finally, the excretory functions of the kidneys and lungs.

A buffer is a substance that resists pH change by absorbing or releasing hydrogen ions (H^+) when acid or base is added to it. The intracellular and extracellular buffers absorb H^+ ions and transport them to the kidneys for elimination. The carbonic acid/bicarbonate system allows H^+ ions to react with bicarbonate to produce carbon dioxide (CO_2) and water and the CO_2 is eliminated by the lungs:

$$H^+ + HCO_3^- \leftrightarrow H_2CO_3 \leftrightarrow CO_2 + H_2O$$
carbonic anhydrase (enzyme)

Carbonic acid (H_2CO_3) continually breaks down to form CO_2 and water, hence this system always tends to move in a rightward direction and, unlike other buffer systems, never gets saturated. But it is easy to see how, for example, a problem with ventilation would quickly lead to a build-up of CO_2, a respiratory acidosis. Uniquely, the components of the carbonic acid/bicarbonate system can be adjusted independently of one another. The kidneys can regulate H^+ ions excretion in the urine and CO_2 levels can be adjusted by changing ventilation. The excretory functions of the lungs and kidneys are connected by carbonic acid so that if one organ becomes overwhelmed, the other can 'help' or 'compensate'.

The lungs have a simple way of regulating CO_2 excretion, but the kidneys have three main ways of excreting H^+ ions:

1 Mainly by regulating the amount of bicarbonate (HCO_3^-) absorbed in the proximal tubule

2 By the reaction $HPO_4^{2-} + H^+ \rightarrow H_2PO_4^-$. The H^+ ions comes from carbonic acid, leaving HCO_3^- which passes into the blood

3 By combining ammonia with H^+ ions from carbonic acid. The resulting ammonium ions cannot pass back into the cells and are excreted.

The kidney produces bicarbonate (HCO_3^-) which reacts with free H^+ ions. This is why the bicarbonate level is low when there is an excess of H^+ ions or a metabolic acidosis.

In summary, the body is continually producing acid, yet at the same time must maintain a narrow pH range in order to function effectively. It does this by means of buffers and then the excretory functions of the lungs (CO_2) and kidneys (H^+). It follows therefore that acid–base disturbances occur when there is a problem with ventilation, a problem with renal function, or an overwhelming acid or base load the body cannot handle.

Some definitions

Before moving on, it is important to understand some important definitions regarding arterial blood gases:

- Acidaemia or alkalaemia: a low or high pH.
- Acidosis: a process which leads to acidaemia (e.g. high $PaCO_2$ or excess H^+ ions (low bicarbonate)).
- Alkalosis: a process which leads to alkalaemia (e.g. low $PaCO_2$ or high bicarbonate).
- Compensation: normal acid–base balance is a normal pH plus a normal $PaCO_2$ and normal bicarbonate. Compensation is when there is a normal pH but the bicarbonate and $PaCO_2$ are abnormal.
- Correction: the restoration of normal pH, $PaCO_2$ and bicarbonate.
- Base excess (BE): this measures how much extra acid or base is in the system as a result of a metabolic problem. It is calculated by measuring the amount of strong acid that has to be added to a sample to produce a pH of 7.4. A minus figure means the sample is already acidotic so no acid had to be added. A plus figure means the sample is alkalotic and acid had to be added. The normal range is -2 to $+2$. A minus BE is often termed a 'base deficit'.
- Actual vs standard bicarbonate: a problem with ventilation would quickly lead to a build-up of CO_2 or a respiratory acidosis. This CO_2 reacts with water to produce H^+ and HCO_3^-, and therefore causes a small and immediate rise in bicarbonate. The *standard* bicarbonate is calculated by the blood gas analyser from the actual bicarbonate, but assuming 37°C and a normal $PaCO_2$ of 5.3 kPa (40 mmHg). Standard bicarbonate therefore reflects the metabolic component of acid–base balance, as opposed to any changes in bicarbonate that have occurred as a result of a respiratory problem. Some

blood gas machines only report the actual bicarbonate, in which case you should use the BE to examine the metabolic component of acid–base balance. Otherwise, the *standard* bicarbonate and BE are interchangeable. *Note*: If you do not like equations, skip the box below.

Box 3.1 pH and the Henderson–Hasselbach equation

Everyone has heard of the Henderson–Hasselbach equation, but what is it? H^+ ions are difficult to measure as there are literally billions of them. We use pH instead, which, simply put, is the negative logarithm of the H^+ ion concentration in moles:

$$pH = -log[H^+]$$

When carbonic (H_2CO_3) acid dissociates:

$$H_2CO_3 \leftrightarrow H^+ + HCO_3^-$$

the product of $[H^+]$ and $[HCO_3^-]$ divided by $[H_2CO_3]$ remains constant. Put in equation form:

$$Ka = \frac{[H^+][HCO_3^-]}{[H_2CO_3]}$$

Ka is the dissociation constant. pKa is like pH, it is the negative logarithm of Ka. The Henderson–Hasselbach equation puts the pH and the dissociation equations together, and describes the relationship between pH and the molal concentrations of the dissociated and undissociated form of carbonic acid:

$$pH = pKa + log\frac{[HCO_3^-]}{[H_2CO_3]}$$

Since $[H_2CO_3]$ is related to $PaCO_2$, a simplified version is:

$$pH \propto \frac{[HCO_3^-]}{PaCO_2}$$

This simple relationship can be used to check the consistency of arterial blood gas data. If we know that pH (or the concentration of H^+ ions) is related to the ratio of HCO_3^- and $PaCO_2$, it should be easy to check whether a blood gas result is 'real' or not, or the result of laboratory error (see Appendix at the end of this chapter).

Common causes of acid–base disturbances

As previously mentioned, acid–base disturbances occur when there is:
- A problem with ventilation
- A problem with renal function
- An overwhelming acid or base load the body cannot handle.

Respiratory acidosis

Respiratory acidosis is caused by acute or chronic alveolar hypoventilation. The causes are described in Chapter 2 and include upper or lower airway obstruction, reduced lung compliance from infection, oedema, trauma or obesity and anything that causes respiratory muscle weakness, including fatigue.

In an acute respiratory acidosis, cellular buffering is effective within minutes to hours. Renal compensation takes 3–5 days to be fully effective. We know from human volunteer studies [1] by how much the standard bicarbonate rises as part of the compensatory response. Although doctors do not frequently use these figures in everyday practice, having a rough idea is nevertheless useful (see Fig. 3.1).

Respiratory alkalosis

Respiratory alkalosis is caused by alveolar hyperventilation, the opposite of respiratory acidosis, and is nearly always accompanied by an increased respiratory rate. Again, renal compensation takes up to 5 days to be fully effective, by excreting bicarbonate in the urine and retaining H^+ ions. When asked what causes hyperventilation, junior doctors invariably reply 'hysteria'. In fact, hyperventilation is a sign, not a diagnosis and has many causes:
- Lung causes: bronchospasm, hypoxaemia, pulmonary embolism, pneumonia, pneumothorax, pulmonary oedema

	Primary change	Compensatory response
Metabolic acidosis	↓ $[HCO_3^-]$	For every 1 mmol/l fall in $[HCO_3^-]$, $PaCO_2$ falls by 0.15 kPa (1.2 mmHg)
Metabolic alkalosis	↑ $[HCO_3^-]$	For every 1 mmol/l rise in $[HCO_3^-]$, $PaCO_2$ rises by 0.01 kPa (0.7 mmHg)
Acute respiratory acidosis	↑ $PaCO_2$	For every 1.3 kPa (10 mmHg) rise in $PaCO_2$, $[HCO_3^-]$ rises by 1 mmol/l
Chronic respiratory acidosis	↑ $PaCO_2$	For every 1.3 kPa (10 mmHg) rise in $PaCO_2$, $[HCO_3^-]$ rises by 3.5 mmol/l
Acute respiratory alkalosis	↓ $PaCO_2$	For every 1.3 kPa (10 mmHg) fall in $PaCO_2$, $[HCO_3^-]$ falls by 2 mmol/l
Chronic respiratory alkalosis	↓ $PaCO_2$	For every 1.3 kPa (10 mmHg) fall in $PaCO_2$, $[HCO_3^-]$ falls by 4 mmol/l

Figure 3.1 Renal and respiratory compensation. Reproduced with permission from McGraw-Hill Publishers [1].

- Central nervous system causes: meningitis/encephalitis, raised intracranial pressure, stroke, cerebral haemorrhage
- Metabolic causes: fever, hyperthyroidism
- Drugs (e.g. salicylate poisoning)
- Psychogenic causes: pain, anxiety.

Metabolic acidosis

Metabolic acidosis most commonly arises from an overwhelming acid load. Respiratory compensation occurs within minutes. Maximal compensation occurs within 12–24 h, but respiratory compensation is limited by the work involved in breathing and the systemic effects of a low CO_2 (mainly cerebral vasoconstriction). It is unusual for the body to be able to fully compensate for a metabolic acidosis.

There are many potential causes of a metabolic acidosis, so it is important to subdivide these into metabolic acidosis with an increased anion gap or metabolic acidosis with a normal anion gap. In general, a metabolic acidosis with an increased anion gap is caused by the body gaining acid, whereas a metabolic acidosis with a normal anion gap is caused by the body losing base.

The anion gap

Blood tests measure most cations (positively charged molecules) but only a few anions (negatively charged molecules). Anions and cations are equal in the human body, but if all the measured cations and anions are added together there would be a gap – this reflects the concentration of those anions not measured, mainly plasma proteins. This is called the anion gap and is calculated from a blood sample:

(sodium + potassium) − (chloride + bicarbonate)

The normal range for the anion gap is 15–20 mmol/l, but this varies from one laboratory to another and should be adjusted downwards in patients with a low albumin (by 2.5 mmol/l for every 1 g/dl fall in plasma albumin). Similarly, a fall in any unmeasured cations (e.g. calcium or magnesium) may produce a spurious increase in the anion gap.

Some patients may have more than one reason to have a metabolic acidosis (e.g. diarrhoea leading to loss of bicarbonate plus severe sepsis and hypoperfusion). Many blood gas machines calculate the anion gap but if not, it should always be calculated when there is a metabolic acidosis, as this helps to narrow down the cause. The base deficit is known to correlate with mortality [2]. A severe metabolic acidosis indicates critical illness.

Metabolic acidosis with an increased anion gap

In a metabolic acidosis with an increased anion gap, the body has gained acid through:
- Ingestion
- The body's own production
- An inability to excrete it

Common clinical causes are:
- Ingestion: salicylate, methanol/ethylene glycol, tricyclic antidepressant poisoning
- Lactic acidosis type A (anaerobic tissue metabolism): any condition causing tissue hypoperfusion, either global (e.g. shock, cardiac arrest) or local (e.g. intra-abdominal ischaemia)
- Lactic acidosis type B (liver dysfunction): reduced lactate metabolism in liver failure, metformin (rare)
- Ketoacidosis: insulin deficiency (diabetic ketoacidosis), starvation
- Renal failure
- Massive rhabdomyolysis (damaged cells release H^+ ions and organic anions).

Metabolic acidosis with a normal anion gap
In a metabolic acidosis with a normal anion gap, bicarbonate is lost via the kidneys or the gastrointestinal tract. Occasionally reduced renal H^+ ions excretion is the cause. A normal anion gap metabolic acidosis is sometimes also called 'hyperchloraemic acidosis'. Common clinical causes are:
- Renal tubular acidosis
- Diarrhoea, fistula or ileostomy
- Acetazolomide therapy.

Overall, the most common cause of a metabolic acidosis in hospital is tissue hypoperfusion. Oxygen and fluid resuscitation are important aspects of treatment, as well as treatment of the underlying cause.

Metabolic alkalosis
Metabolic alkalosis is the least well known of the acid–base disturbances. It can be divided into two groups: *saline responsive* and *saline unresponsive*. Saline responsive metabolic alkalosis is the most common and occurs with volume contraction (e.g. vomiting or diuretic use). Gastric outflow obstruction is a well-known cause of 'hypokalaemic hypochloraemic metabolic alkalosis'. Excessive vomiting or nasogastric suction leads to loss of hydrochloric acid, but the decline in glomerular filtration rate which accompanies this perpetuates the metabolic alkalosis. The kidneys try to reabsorb chloride (hence the urine levels are low), but there is less of it from loss of hydrochloric acid, so the only available anion to be reabsorbed is bicarbonate. Metabolic alkalosis is often associated with hypokalaemia, due to secondary hyperaldosteronism from volume depletion.

Another relatively common cause of saline responsive metabolic alkalosis is when hypercapnia is corrected quickly by mechanical ventilation. Post-hypercapnia alkalosis occurs because a high $PaCO_2$ directly affects the proximal tubules and decreases sodium chloride reabsorption leading to volume depletion. If chronic hypercapnia is corrected rapidly with mechanical ventilation, metabolic alkalosis ensues because there is already a high bicarbonate and the kidney needs time to excrete it. The pH change causes a shift in potassium with resulting hypokalaemia and sometimes cardiac arrhythmias.

Saline unresponsive metabolic alkalosis occurs due to renal problems:
- With high BP: excess mineralocorticoid (exogenous or endogenous)
- With normal BP: severe low potassium, high calcium

Mini-tutorial: The use of i.v. sodium bicarbonate in metabolic acidosis

HCO_3^- as sodium bicarbonate may be administered i.v. to raise blood pH in severe metabolic acidosis but this poses several problems. It increases the formation of CO_2 which passes readily into cells (unlike HCO_3^-) and this worsens intracellular acidosis. The oxygen-dissociation curve is shifted to the left by alkalosis leading to impaired oxygen delivery to the tissues. Sodium bicarbonate contains a significant sodium load and because 8.4% solution is hypertonic, the increase in plasma osmolality can lead to vasodilatation and hypotension. Tissue necrosis can result from extravasation from the cannula. Some patients with airway or ventilation problems may need mechanical ventilation to counter the increased CO_2 production caused by an infusion of sodium bicarbonate. Many of the causes of metabolic acidosis respond to restoration of intravascular volume and tissue perfusion with oxygen, i.v. fluids and treatment of the underlying cause. For these reasons, routine i.v. sodium bicarbonate is not used in a metabolic acidosis. It tends to be reserved for specific conditions, for example tricyclic poisoning (when it acts as an antidote), treatment of hyperkalaemia and some cases of renal failure. It may also be used in other situations, but only by experts: 8.4% sodium bicarbonate = 1 mmol/ml of sodium or bicarbonate.

- High-dose penicillin therapy
- Ingestion of exogenous alkali with a low glomerular filtration rate

A summary of the changes in pH, $PaCO_2$ and standard bicarbonate in different acid–base disturbances is shown in Fig. 3.2.

Interpreting an arterial blood gas report

There are a few simple rules when looking at an arterial blood gas report:
- Always consider the clinical situation
- An abnormal pH indicates the primary acid–base problem
- The body never overcompensates
- Mixed acid–base disturbances are common in clinical practice.

Any test has to be interpreted only in the light of the clinical situation. A normal blood gas result might be reassuring, but not, for example, if the patient has severe asthma, where a 'normal' $PaCO_2$ level would be extremely worrying. The body's compensatory mechanisms only aim to bring the pH towards normal and never swing like a pendulum in the opposite direction. So a low pH with a high $PaCO_2$ and high standard bicarbonate is always a respiratory acidosis and never an overcompensated metabolic alkalosis. These principles will be easily seen as you work through the case histories at the end of this chapter. Many doctors miss vital information when interpreting arterial blood gas reports because they do not use a systematic method of doing so.

There are five steps in interpreting an arterial blood gas report:
1 Look at the pH first
2 Look at the $PaCO_2$ and the standard bicarbonate (or BE) to see whether this is a respiratory or a metabolic problem, or both

	pH	PaCO$_2$	St bicarbonate/BE	Compensatory response
Respiratory acidosis	Low	High	Normal	St bicarbonate rises
Metabolic acidosis	Low	Normal	Low	PaCO$_2$ falls
Respiratory alkalosis	High	Low	Normal	St bicarbonate falls
Metabolic alkalosis	High	Normal	High	PaCO$_2$ rises

Figure 3.2 Changes in pH, PaCO$_2$ and standard bicarbonate in different acid–base disturbances.

3 Check the appropriateness of any compensation. For example, in a metabolic acidosis you would expect the PaCO$_2$ to be low. If the PaCO$_2$ is normal this indicates a 'hidden' respiratory acidosis as well
4 Calculate the anion gap if there is a metabolic acidosis
5 Finally, look at the PaO$_2$ and compare it to the inspired oxygen concentration (more on this in Chapter 4).

Why arterial blood gases are an important test in critical illness

Arterial blood gas analysis can be performed quickly and gives the following useful information:
- A measure of oxygenation (PaO$_2$)
- A measure of ventilation (PaCO$_2$)
- A measure of perfusion (standard bicarbonate or BE).
In other words, a measure of A, B and C, which is why it is an extremely useful test in the management of a critically ill patient.

Key points – acid–base balance

- The body maintains a narrow pH range using buffers and then the excretory functions of the lungs and kidneys.
- Acid–base disturbances occur when there is a problem with ventilation, a problem with renal function, or an overwhelming acid or base load the body cannot handle.
- Use the five steps outlined above when interpreting an arterial blood gas report so that important information is not missed.
- Arterial blood gas analysis is an important test in critical illness.

Self-assessment: case histories

Normal values: pH 7.35–7.45, PaCO$_2$ 4.5–6.0 (35–46 mmHg), PaO$_2$ 11–14.5 kPa (83–108 mmHg), BE −2 to + 2, st bicarbonate 22–28 mmol/l.
1 A 65-year-old man with chronic obstructive pulmonary disease (COPD) comes to the emergency department with shortness of breath. His arterial

blood gases on air show: pH 7.29, $PaCO_2$ 8.5 kPa (65.3 mmHg), st bicarbonate 30.5 mmol/l, BE +4, PaO_2 8.0 kPa (62 mmHg). What is the acid–base disturbance and what is your management?

2 A 60-year-old ex-miner with COPD is admitted with shortness of breath. His arterial blood gases on air show: pH 7.36, $PaCO_2$ 9.0 kPa (65.3 mmHg), st bicarbonate 35 mmol/l, BE +6, PaO_2 6.0 kPa (46.1 mmHg). What is the acid–base disturbance and what is your management?

3 A 24-year-old man with epilepsy comes to hospital in tonic–clonic status epilepticus. He is given i.v. Lorazepam. Arterial blood gases on 10 l/min oxygen via reservoir bag mask show: pH 7.05, $PaCO_2$ 8.0 (61.5 mmHg), standard bicarbonate 16 mmol/l, BE −8, PaO_2 15 kPa (115 mmHg). His other results are sodium 140 mmol/l, potassium 4 mmol/l and chloride 98 mmol/l. What is his acid–base status and why? What is your management?

4 A 44-year-old man comes to the emergency department with pleuritic chest pain and shortness of breath which he has had for a few days. A small pneumothorax is seen on the chest X-ray. His arterial blood gases on 10 l/min oxygen via simple face mask show: pH 7.44, $PaCO_2$ 3.0 (23 mmHg), st bicarbonate 16 mmol/l, BE −8, PaO_2 30.5 kPa (234.6 mmHg). Is there a problem with acid–base balance?

5 A patient is admitted to hospital with breathlessness and arterial blood gases on air show: pH 7.2, $PaCO_2$ 4.1 kPa (31.5 mmHg), st bicarbonate 36 mmol/l, BE +10, PaO_2 7.8 kPa (60 mmHg). Can you explain this?

6 An 80-year-old woman is admitted with abdominal pain. Her vital signs are normal, apart from cool peripheries and a tachycardia. Her arterial blood gases on air show: pH 7.1, $PaCO_2$ 3.5 kPa (30 mmHg), st bicarbonate 8 mmol/l, BE −20, PaO_2 12 kPa (92 mmHg). You review the clinical situation again – she has generalised tenderness in the abdomen but it is soft. Her blood glucose is 6.0 mmol/l (100 mg/dl), her creatinine and liver tests are normal. The chest X-ray is normal. There are reduced bowel sounds. The ECG shows atrial fibrillation. What is the reason for the acid–base disturbance? What is your management?

7 A 30-year-old woman who is 36 weeks pregnant has her arterial blood gases taken on air because of pleuritic chest pain. The results are as follows: pH 7.48, $PaCO_2$ 3.4 kPa (26 mmHg), st bicarbonate 19 mmol/l, BE −4, PaO_2 14 kPa (108 mmHg). What do these blood gases show? Could they indicate a pulmonary embolism?

8 A 45-year-old woman with a history of peptic ulcer disease reports 6 days of persistent vomiting. On examination she has a BP of 100/60 mmHg and looks dehydrated and unwell. Her blood results are as follows: sodium 140 mmol/l, potassium 2.2 mmol/l, chloride 86 mmol/l, venous (actual) bicarbonate 40 mmol/l, urea 29 mmol/l (blood urea nitrogen (BUN) 80 mg/dl), pH 7.5, $PaCO_2$ 6.2 kPa (53 mmHg), PaO_2 14 kPa (107 mmHg), urine pH 5.0, urine sodium 2 mmol/l, urine potassium 21 mmol/l and urine chloride 3 mmol/l. What is the acid–base disturbance? How would you treat this patient? Twenty-four hours after appropriate therapy the venous bicarbonate is 30 mmol/l

and the following urine values are obtained: pH 7.8, sodium 100 mmol/l, potassium 20 mmol/l and chloride 3 mmol/l. How do you account for the high urinary sodium but low urinary chloride concentration?

9 A 50-year-old man is recovering on a surgical ward 10 days after a total colectomy for bowel obstruction. He has type 1 diabetes and is on i.v. insulin. His ileostomy is working normally. His vital signs are: BP 150/70 mmHg, respiratory rate 16/min, SpO_2 98% on air, urine output 1200 ml per day, temperature normal and he is well perfused. The surgical team are concerned about his persistently high potassium (which was noted pre-operatively as well) and metabolic acidosis. His blood results are: sodium 130 mmol/l, potassium 6.5 mmol/l, urea 14 mmol/l (BUN 39 mg/dl), creatinine 180 μmol/l (2.16 mg/dl), chloride 109 mmol/l, normal synacthen test and albumin. He is known to have diabetic nephropathy and is on Ramipril. His usual creatinine is 180 μmol/l. His arterial blood gases on air show: pH 7.31, $PaCO_2$ 4.0 kPa (27 mmHg), st bicarbonate 15 mmol/l, BE −8, PaO_2 14 kPa (108 mmHg). The surgical team are wondering whether this persisting metabolic acidosis means that there is an intra-abdominal problem, although a recent abdominal CT scan was normal. What is your advice?

10 Match the clinical history with the appropriate arterial blood gas values:

	pH	$PaCO_2$	St bicarbonate (mmol/l)
a	7.39	8.45 kPa (65 mmHg)	37
b	7.27	7.8 kPa (60 mmHg)	26
c	7.35	7.8 kPa (60 mmHg)	32

- A severely obese 24-year-old man
- A 56-year-old lady with COPD who has been started on a diuretic for peripheral oedema, resulting in a 3 kg weight loss
- A 14-year-old girl with a severe asthma attack.

Self-assessment: discussion

1 There is an acidaemia (low pH) due to a high $PaCO_2$ – a respiratory acidosis. The standard bicarbonate is just above normal. The PaO_2 is low. Management starts with assessment and treatment of airway, breathing and circulation (ABC). Medical treatment of an exacerbation of COPD includes controlled oxygen therapy, nebulised salbutamol, steroids, antibiotics if necessary, i.v. aminophylline in some cases and non-invasive ventilation if the respiratory acidosis does not resolve quickly [3].

2 There is a normal pH with a high $PaCO_2$ (respiratory acidosis) and a high st bicarbonate (metabolic alkalosis). Which came first? The clinical history

and the low-ish pH point towards this being a respiratory acidosis, compensated for by a raise in st bicarbonate (renal compensation). This is a chronic or compensated respiratory acidosis. If the pH fell further due to a rise in $PaCO_2$, you could call this an 'acute on chronic respiratory acidosis' which would look like this: pH 7.17, $PaCO_2$ 14.6 kPa (109 mmHg), standard bicarbonate 39 mmol/l, BE +7.6, PaO_2 6.0 kPa (46.1 mmHg). Management would be the same as for case number 1, but note that non-invasive ventilation is only indicated when the pH falls below 7.35 due to a rise in $PaCO_2$.

3 There is an acidaemia (low pH) due to a high $PaCO_2$ and a low st bicarbonate – a mixed respiratory and metabolic acidosis. The PaO_2 is low in relation to the inspired oxygen concentration. The high $PaCO_2$ is likely to be due to airway obstruction and the respiratory depressant effects of i.v. benzodiazepines. This can be deduced because there is such a large difference between the inspired oxygen concentration (FiO_2) and the PaO_2. Aspiration pneumonia is another possibility. Persistent tonic–clonic seizures cause a lactic acidosis because of anaerobic muscle metabolism. Management starts with assessment and treatment of ABC (followed by disability and examination/planning (DE)). A benzodiazepine aborts 80% seizures in status epilepticus. Lorazepam is the drug of choice because seizures are less likely to relapse compared with diazepam (55% at 24 h compared with 50% at 2 h). Additional therapy is then required to keep seizures away – 15 mg/kg i.v. phenytoin as a slow infusion with cardiac monitoring is the initial treatment. If this fails, consider other diagnoses, further phenytoin and sedation with propofol or barbiturates on the ICU [4].

4 There is a normal pH with a low $PaCO_2$ (respiratory alkalosis) and a low st bicarbonate (metabolic acidosis). Which came first? The history and the high-ish pH point towards this being a respiratory alkalosis, compensated for by a fall in st bicarbonate. This is a compensated respiratory alkalosis. If you saw a similar arterial blood gas in an unwell diabetic, it could be an early (compensated) diabetic ketoacidosis.

5 As you may have guessed, this is an impossible blood gas – the answer is laboratory error!

6 There is an acidaemia (low pH) due to a very low st bicarbonate (metabolic acidosis). The $PaCO_2$ is appropriately low, although it should be lower than this – approximately 2.5 kPa, possibly indicating that she is tiring. The anion gap is not given. The PaO_2 is normal. The presence of atrial fibrillation is a clue to the diagnosis of ischaemic bowel. Intra-abdominal catastrophes are associated with a metabolic acidosis. This case illustrates that an 'acute abdomen' is often soft in the elderly. They commonly show few signs of an inflammatory response because of their less active immune system. Management starts with assessment and treatment of ABC followed by DE – call the surgeon.

7 There is a high pH (alkalaemia) due to a low $PaCO_2$ (respiratory alkalosis). The st bicarbonate is just below normal. The PaO_2 is normal. A respiratory alkalosis is a normal finding in advanced pregnancy [5]. The alveolar–arterial (A-a) gradient is not affected by pregnancy and is normal in this case (see Chapter 4). Arterial blood gases can be normal in peripheral pulmonary emboli and therefore do not add to the management of this case.

8 There is a high pH (alkalaemia) due to a high bicarbonate (metabolic alkalosis). The PaCO$_2$ is just above normal. The PaO$_2$ is normal, assuming she is breathing room air. The potassium and chloride levels are both low. This is the hypokalaemic hypochloraemic metabolic alkalosis seen in prolonged vomiting due to gastric outflow obstruction. The physical findings and low urinary chloride point towards volume depletion. The patient requires i.v. saline (sodium chloride) with potassium. During therapy, volume expansion reduces the need for sodium reabsorption, hence the high levels in the urine. The discrepancy between urinary sodium and chloride is primarily due to urinary bicarbonate excretion. Further saline replacement is necessary for as long as the low urinary chloride persists, since it indicates ongoing chloride and volume depletion.

9 There is a low pH (acidaemia) due to a low st bicarbonate – a metabolic acidosis. The PaCO$_2$ is appropriately low. The anion gap may be calculated as $(130 + 6.5) - (12 + 109) = 15.5$ mmol/l, which is normal. The PaO$_2$ is normal. Common causes of a normal anion gap metabolic acidosis include renal tubular acidosis, diarrhoea, fistula or ileostomy and acetazolomide therapy. In this case, excessive gastrointestinal losses and acetazolomide can be excluded, which leaves a possible renal cause. Renal tubular acidosis is a collection of disorders in which the kidneys either cannot excrete H$^+$ ions or generate bicarbonate. Only one of the renal tubular acidoses is associated with a high serum potassium – type 4, or hyporeninaemic hypoaldosteronism, found in patients with diabetic or hypertensive nephropathy (as in this case) and exacerbated by angiotensin converting enzyme inhibitors, aldosterone blockers, for example spironolactone and nonsteroidal anti-inflammatory drugs. The metabolic acidosis seen in this condition is usually mild, with the st bicarbonate concentration remaining above 15 mmol/l. Treatment usually consists of dietary restriction of potassium and medication, for example oral furosemide.

10 Severe obesity suggests chronic hypercapnia (c). COPD and diuretic therapy suggest chronic hypercapnia with a superimposed metabolic alkalosis (a). A severe asthma attack suggests an acute respiratory acidosis (b).

Appendix: Checking the consistency of arterial blood gas data

H^+ ions concentration is sometimes used instead of pH. A simple conversion between pH 7.2 and 7.5 is that $[H^+] = 80$ minus the two digits after the decimal point. So if the pH is 7.35, then $[H^+]$ is $80 - 35 = 45\,nmol/l$ (see Fig. 3.3).

Earlier in this chapter, Box 3.1 on the Henderson–Hasselbach equation explained that pH is proportional to $[HCO_3^-]/PaCO_2$. Another way of writing this is as follows:

$$[H^+] = Ka \times \frac{PaCO_2}{HCO_3^-} \quad \text{where } Ka \text{ is the dissociation constant}$$

$$\text{or } [H^+] = 181 \times \frac{PaCO_2}{HCO_3^-} \quad \text{in kPa (or } 24 \times PaCO_2 \text{ in mmHg)}$$

The following arterial blood gas analysis: pH 7.25, $PaCO_2$ 4.5 kPa (35 mmHg), st bicarbonate 14.8 mmol/l, PaO_2 8.0 kPa (61 mmHg) shows a metabolic acidosis. A pH of $7.25 = [H^+]$ of 55 nmol/l. Do the figures add up?

$$181 \times \frac{4.5}{14.8} = 55$$

Yes, a $PaCO_2$ of 4.5 kPa with a st bicarbonate of 14.8 would give a $[H^+]$ of 55 nmol/l. You may find this simple calculation useful when checking for laboratory error, or making up arterial blood gases for teaching material.

pH	$[H^+]$ (nmol/l)
7.6	26
7.5	32
7.4	40
7.3	50
7.2	63
7.1	80
7.0	100
6.9	125
6.8	160

Figure 3.3 pH and equivalent $[H^+]$.

References

1. Burton David Rose and Theodore W Post. Introduction to simple and mixed acid–base disorders. In: Clinical Physiology of Acid–Base and Electrolyte Disorders 5th edn. McGraw-Hill, New York, 2001.
2. Whitehead MA, Puthucheary Z and Rhodes A. The recognition of a sick patient. *Clinical Medicine* 2002; **2(2)**: 95–98.
3. Christopher M Ball and Robert S Phillips. Exacerbation of chronic obstructive pulmonary disease. In: *Evidence-Based On Call Acute Medicine*. Churchill Livingstone, London, 2001.
4. Mark Manford. Status epilepticus. In: *Practical Guide to Epilepsy*. Butterworth Heinemann, Burlington, MA, USA, 2003.
5. Girling JC. Management of medical emergencies in pregnancy. *CPD Journal Acute Medicine* 2002; **1(3)**: 96–100.

Further resource

• Driscoll P, Brown T, Gwinnutt C and Wardle T. *A Simple Guide to Blood Gas Analysis*. BMJ Publishing, London, 1997.

CHAPTER 4
Respiratory failure

By the end of this chapter you will be able to:
- Understand basic pulmonary physiology
- Understand the mechanisms of respiratory failure
- Know when respiratory support is indicated
- Know which type of respiratory support to use
- Understand the effects of mechanical ventilation
- Apply this to your clinical practice

Basic pulmonary physiology

The main function of the respiratory system is to supply oxygenated blood and remove carbon dioxide. This process is achieved by:
- Ventilation: the delivery and removal of gas to and from the alveoli.
- Gas exchange: oxygen and carbon dioxide (CO_2) cross the alveolar–capillary wall by diffusion.
- Circulation: oxygen is transported from the lungs to the cells and carbon dioxide is transported from the cells to the lungs. The concept of oxygen delivery has been outlined in Chapter 2 and will not be discussed further here.

When it comes to respiratory failure, there are two types: failure to ventilate and failure to oxygenate. An understanding of basic pulmonary physiology is important in understanding why respiratory failure occurs.

Ventilation
During inspiration, the volume of the thoracic cavity increases, due to contraction of the diaphragm and movement of the ribs, and air is actively drawn into the lung. Beyond the terminal bronchioles is the respiratory zone, where the surface area of the lung is huge and diffusion of gas occurs. The lung is elastic and returns passively to its pre-inspiratory volume on expiration. The lung is also very compliant – a normal breath requires only 3 cmH_2O of pressure.

A normal breath (500 ml) is only a small proportion of total lung volume, shown diagrammatically in Fig. 4.1. Of each 500 ml inhaled, 150 ml stays in the anatomical deadspace and does not take part in gas exchange. Most of the rest of the gas which enters the respiratory zone takes part in *alveolar* ventilation, but around 5% does not due to normal ventilation–perfusion (V/Q) mismatch,

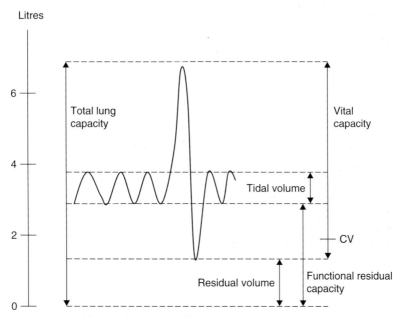

Figure 4.1 Normal lung volumes. The closing volume (CV) is the volume at which the dependent airways begin to collapse, or close. It is normally about 10% of the vital capacity and increases to about 40% by the age of 65 years.

and this is called the alveolar deadspace. The anatomical plus alveolar deadspace is called the physiological deadspace. In health, the anatomical and physiological deadspaces are almost the same.

V/Q mismatch can increase in disease. If ventilation is reduced to a part of the lung and blood flow remains unchanged, alveolar O_2 will fall and CO_2 will rise in that area, approaching the values of venous blood. If blood flow is obstructed to a part of the lung and ventilation remains unchanged, alveolar O_2 will rise and CO_2 will fall in that area, approaching the values of inspired air. The V/Q ratio therefore lies along a continuum, ranging from zero (perfusion but no ventilation, i.e. shunt) to infinity (ventilation but no perfusion, i.e. increased deadspace).

When PaO_2 falls and $PaCO_2$ rises due to V/Q mismatch, normal people increase their overall alveolar ventilation to compensate. This corrects the hypercapnia but only partially the hypoxaemia due to the different shapes of the O_2 and CO_2 dissociation curves.

The alveolar–arterial (A-a) gradient is a measure of V/Q mismatch and is discussed later.

The mechanics of ventilation are complex. Surfactant plays an important role in the elastic properties of the lung (and is depleted in acute respiratory distress syndrome). The lungs tend to recoil while the thoracic cage tends to expand slightly. This creates a negative intrapleural pressure, which increases during

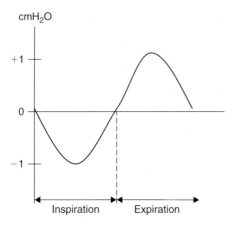

Inspiration   Expiration

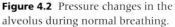

Figure 4.2 Pressure changes in the alveolus during normal breathing.

inspiration, because as the lung expands, its elastic recoil increases. Fig. 4.2 shows the pressure changes which occur in the alveolus during normal breathing.

Ventilation is controlled in the brainstem respiratory centres, with input from the cortex (voluntary control). The muscles which affect ventilation are the diaphragm, intercostals, abdominal muscles and the accessory muscles (e.g. sternomastoids). Ventilation is sensed by central and peripheral chemoreceptors, and other receptors in the lungs. Normally, $PaCO_2$ is the most important factor in the control of ventilation but the sensitivity to changes in $PaCO_2$ is reduced by sleep, older age and airway resistance (e.g. in chronic obstructive pulmonary disease (COPD)). Other factors which increase ventilation include hypoxaemia, low arterial pH and situations which increase oxygen demand (e.g. sepsis).

Oxygenation

Oxygen tension in the air is around 20 kPa (154 mmHg) at sea level, falling to around 0.5 kPa (3.8 mmHg) in the mitochondria. This gradient is known as the 'oxygen cascade' (illustrated in Fig. 4.3). Therefore, an interruption at any point along this cascade can cause hypoxia (e.g. high altitude, upper or lower airway obstruction, alveolar problems, abnormal haemoglobins, circulatory failure or mitochondrial poisoning).

If a patient is breathing 60% oxygen and his/her PaO_2 is 13 kPa (100 mmHg), it can be seen that there is a significant problem with gas exchange – the 'normal' value of 13 kPa is not normal at all in the context of a high inspired oxygen concentration (F_iO_2). With normal lungs, the predicted PaO_2 is roughly 10 kPa (75 mmHg) below the F_iO_2. Problems with gas exchange occur at the alveolar–arterial (A-a) step of the oxygen cascade (D to E in Fig. 4.3). Normal people have a small A-a difference because the bronchial veins of the lung and Thebesian veins of the heart carry unsaturated blood directly to the left ventricle, bypassing the alveoli. Large differences are always due to pathology.

In the example above, one can see the difference between F_iO_2 and PaO_2 without a calculation. However, the difference between alveolar and arterial oxygen (the A-a gradient) can be measured using the alveolar gas equation.

Oxygen partial pressure (vertical) in different parts of the body (horizontal)

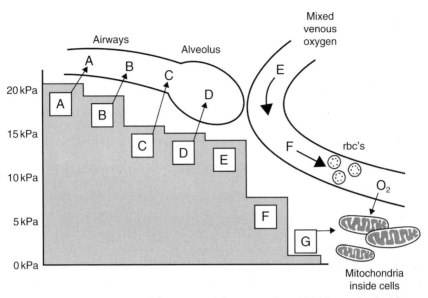

Figure 4.3 The oxygen cascade. A: inspired dry gas; B: humidified; C: mixed with expired gas; D: alveolar ventilation + oxygen consumption; E: venous mixing + V/Q mismatch; F: capillary blood; G: mitochondria.

Oxygen leaves the alveolus in exchange for carbon dioxide. Arterial and alveolar PCO_2 are virtually the same. If we know the composition of inspired gas and the respiratory exchange ratio (R), then the alveolar oxygen concentration can be calculated. (The respiratory exchange ratio allows for metabolism by the tissues.) To convert F_iO_2 into the *partial pressure* of inspired O_2, we have to adjust for barometric pressure, water vapour pressure and temperature. Assuming sea level (101 kPa or 760 mmHg), inspired air which is 100% humidified (water vapour pressure 6 kPa or 47 mmHg) and 37°C, the alveolar gas equation is as follows:

$$P_AO_2 = F_iO_2 (P_B - P_AH_2O) - P_ACO_2/0.8$$

P_AO_2: alveolar PO_2
F_iO_2: fraction of inspired oxygen
P_B: barometric pressure of 101 kPa
P_AH_2O: alveolar partial pressure of water of 6 kPa
P_ACO_2: alveolar PCO_2
0.8: the respiratory exchange ratio (or respiratory quotient).

Once P_AO_2 has been estimated, the A-a gradient is calculated as $P_AO_2 - PaO_2$. A normal A-a gradient is up to 2 kPa (15 mmHg) or 4 kPa (30 mmHg) in smokers and the elderly.

For example, a person breathing air with a PaO_2 of 12.0 kPa and a $PaCO_2$ of 5.0 kPa has an A-a gradient as follows:

$$P_AO_2 = F_iO_2 (P_B - P_AH_2O) - P_ACO_2/0.8$$

$$P_AO_2 = 0.21 \times 95 - 5/0.8$$

When calculating the A-a gradient on air, 0.21×95 is often shortened to 20.

$$20 - 5/0.8 = 13.75$$

The A-a gradient is therefore $13.75 - 12 = 1.75$ kPa.

The calculation of the A-a gradient illustrates the importance of always documenting the inspired oxygen concentration on an arterial blood gas report, otherwise problems with oxygenation may not be detected. Some applications of the A-a gradient are illustrated in the case histories at the end of this chapter.

The mechanisms of respiratory failure

Respiratory failure is said to be present when there is PaO_2 of <8.0 kPa (60 mmHg), when breathing air at sea level without intracardiac shunting. It occurs with or without a high $PaCO_2$.

Traditionally, respiratory failure is divided into type 1 and type 2, but these are not practical terms and it is better to think instead of:
• Failure to ventilate
• Failure to oxygenate
• Failure to both ventilate and oxygenate.

Failure to ventilate

V/Q mismatch causes a high $PaCO_2$, as mentioned earlier. But hypercapnic respiratory failure occurs when the patient cannot compensate for a high $PaCO_2$ by increasing overall alveolar ventilation and this usually occurs in conditions which cause alveolar hypoventilation.

Fig. 2.8 illustrated how respiratory muscle load and respiratory muscle strength can be affected by disease and an imbalance leads to alveolar hypoventilation. To recap, respiratory muscle load is increased by increased resistance (e.g. upper or lower airway obstruction), reduced compliance (e.g. infection, oedema, rib fractures or obesity) and increased respiratory rate (RR). Respiratory muscle strength can be reduced by a problem in any part of the neuro-respiratory pathway: motor neurone disease, Guillain–Barré syndrome, myasthenia gravis or electrolyte abnormalities (low potassium, magnesium, phosphate or calcium). Drugs which act on the respiratory centre, such as morphine, reduce total ventilation.

Oxygen therapy corrects hypoxaemia which occurs as a result of V/Q mismatch or alveolar hypoventilation.

Failure to oxygenate

Although there are many potential causes of hypoxaemia, as illustrated by the oxygen cascade, the most common causes of failure to oxygenate are:

- V/Q mismatch
- Intrapulmonary shunt
- Diffusion problems.

V/Q mismatch

If the airways are impaired by the presence of secretions or narrowed by bronchoconstriction, that segment will be perfused but only partially ventilated. The resulting V/Q mismatch will result in hypoxaemia and hypercapnia. The patient will increase his/her overall alveolar ventilation to compensate. Giving supplemental oxygen will cause the PaO_2 to increase.

Intrapulmonary shunt

If the airways are totally filled with fluid or collapsed, that segment will be perfused but not ventilated at all (see Fig. 4.4). Mixed venous blood is shunted across it. Increasing the inspired oxygen in the presence of a moderate to severe shunt will not improve PaO_2. Intrapulmonary shunting as a cause of hypoxaemia is observed in pneumonia and atelectasis.

V/Q mismatch and intrapulmonary shunting can often be distinguished by the response of the patient to supplemental oxygen. With a large shunt, hypoxaemia cannot be abolished even by giving the patient high-concentration oxygen. Small reductions in inspired oxygen may lead to a large reduction in PaO_2 because of the relatively steep part of the oxygen dissociation curve (see Fig. 2.11).

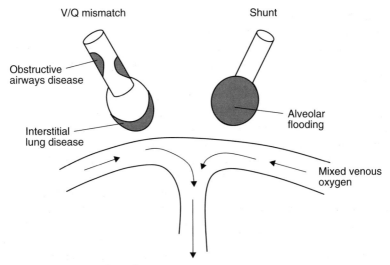

Figure 4.4 V/Q mismatch vs shunt.

Diffusion problems

Some conditions affect the blood–gas barrier (e.g. fibrosis), which is normally extremely thin, leading to ineffective diffusion of gas. The response to supplemental oxygen reduces with increasing severity of disease.

With V/Q mismatch, intrapulmonary shunt and diffusion problems, there is adequate ventilation but inadequate gas exchange and therefore a low PaO_2 with a normal or low $PaCO_2$ is seen.

Failure to both ventilate and oxygenate

Post-operative respiratory failure is an example of a situation where problems with gas exchange are accompanied by hypoventilation, leading to hypoxaemia (despite oxygen therapy) as well as hypercapnia. In post-operative respiratory failure, the hypoxaemia is caused by infection and atelectasis due to a combination of supine position, the effects of general anaesthesia and pain. A reduction in functional residual capacity below closing volume also contributes leading to airway collapse in the dependent parts of the lung (see Fig. 4.1). The hypercapnia is caused by excessive load from reduced compliance and increased minute volume in combination with opiates which depress ventilation. At-risk patients are those with pre-existing lung disease, who are obese or who have upper abdominal or thoracic surgery. Box 4.1 outlines the measures to prevent post-operative respiratory failure.

Respiratory support

Ideally, patients with acute respiratory failure which does not rapidly reverse with medical therapy should be admitted to a respiratory care unit or other level 2–3 facility. Hypoxaemia is the most life-threatening facet of respiratory failure. The goal of treatment is to ensure adequate oxygen delivery to the tissues which is generally achieved with a PaO_2 of at least 8.0 kPa (60 mmHg) or SpO_2 of at least 93%. However, patients with chronic respiratory failure require different therapeutic targets than patients with previously normal lungs. One would not necessarily aim for normal values in these patients.

Box 4.1 Preventing post-operative respiratory failure

- Identify high-risk patients pre-operatively: pre-existing lung disease, upper abdominal or thoracic surgery, smokers (impaired ciliary transport), obesity
- Use regional analgesia if possible
- Early post-operative chest physiotherapy
- Humidified oxygen
- Avoid use of drugs which may depress ventilation
- Early identification of pneumonia
- Early use of CPAP

Apart from oxygen therapy (see Chapter 2) and treatment of the underlying cause, various forms of respiratory support are used in the treatment of respiratory failure. There are two main types of respiratory support: non-invasive and invasive. Non-invasive respiratory support consists of either bilevel positive airway pressure (BiPAP) or continuous positive airway pressure (CPAP), administered via a tight-fitting mask. Invasive respiratory support, on the other hand, requires endotracheal intubation and comes in several different modes.

'Respiratory support' does not necessarily mean mechanical ventilation. For example, CPAP is not ventilation, as will be explained later. The ABCDE (airway, breathing, circulation, disability, examination and planning) approach is still important, and should be used to assess and manage any patient with respiratory failure (see Box 4.2).

Respiratory support is indicated when:
- There is a failure to oxygenate or ventilate despite medical therapy
- There is unacceptable respiratory fatigue
- There are non-respiratory indications for tracheal intubation and ventilation (e.g. the need for airway protection).

Once a decision has been made that a patient needs respiratory support, the next question is, which type? Failure to ventilate is treated by manoeuvres

---

Box 4.2 Approach to the patient with respiratory failure

Action

A   Assess and treat any upper airway obstruction
     Administer oxygen

B   *Look* at the chest: assess rate, depth and symmetry
     Measure SpO_2
     Quickly listen with a stethoscope (for air entry, wheeze, crackles)
     You may need to use a bag and mask if the patient has inadequate ventilation
     Treat wheeze, pneumothorax, fluid, collapse, infection etc
     Is a physiotherapist needed?

C   Fluid challenge(s) or rehydration may be needed
     Vasoactive drugs may be needed if severe sepsis is also present (see Chapter 6)

D   Assess conscious level as this affects treatment options

E   Are ABCD stable? If not, go back to the top and call for help
     Arterial blood gases
     Gather more information (e.g. usual lung function)
     Decide if and what type of respiratory support is needed
     Make ICU and cardio-pulmonary resuscitation (CPR) decisions now
     Do not move an unstable patient without the right monitoring equipment and staff
     Call a senior colleague (if not already called)

designed to increase alveolar minute ventilation by increasing the depth and
rate of breathing. Failure to oxygenate, however, is treated by restoring and
maintaining lung volumes using alveolar recruitment manoeuvres such as
the application of a positive end-expiratory pressure (PEEP or CPAP). Fig. 4.5
summarises the different types of respiratory support.

There is considerable evidence available as to what works best in different
clinical situations [1]. This information is important. For example, there is no
evidence that 'trying' non-invasive ventilation (NIV) in a young person with
life-threatening asthma is of any benefit. The first-line methods of respiratory
support for different conditions are shown in Fig. 4.6.

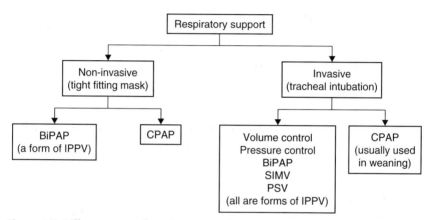

Figure 4.5 Different types of respiratory support. BiPAP: bilevel positive pressure
ventilation; IPPV: intermittent positive pressure ventilation; CPAP: continuous
positive airway pressure; SIMV: synchronised intermittent mandatory ventilation;
PSV: pressure support ventilation.

Tracheal intubation	Non-invasive ventilation (NIV/BiPAP)	Non-invasive CPAP
• Asthma • ARDS (acute respiratory distress syndrome) • Severe respiratory acidosis causing pH <7.25 • Any cause with impaired conscious level • Pneumonia*	• COPD with respiratory acidosis causing pH 7.25–7.35 • Decompensated sleep apnoea • Acute on chronic hypercapnic respiratory failure due to chest wall deformity or neuromuscular disease	• Acute cardiogenic pulmonary oedema • Hypoxaemia in chest trauma/atelectasis

Figure 4.6 First-line methods of respiratory support for different conditions. *If NIV or
CPAP is used as a trial of treatment in pneumonia in patients without COPD or post-
operative respiratory failure, this should be done on an ICU with close monitoring and
rapid access to intubation. Patients with excessive secretions may also require tracheal
intubation.

Non-invasive respiratory support

Non-invasive respiratory support will be more familiar to people who do not work on an intensive care unit (ICU). BiPAP and CPAP are the two main types of non-invasive respiratory support. Non-invasive BiPAP is also referred to as NIV. The ventilator cycles between two different pressures triggered by the patient's own breathing, the higher inspiratory positive airway pressure (IPAP) and the lower expiratory positive airway pressure (EPAP). In CPAP a single positive pressure is applied throughout the patient's respiratory cycle. The difference between non-invasive BiPAP and CPAP is shown in Fig. 4.7.

Non-invasive respiratory support is contraindicated in:
- Recent facial or upper airway surgery, facial burns or trauma
- Vomiting
- Recent upper gastrointestinal surgery or bowel obstruction
- Inability to protect own airway
- Copious respiratory secretions
- Other organ system failure (e.g. haemodynamic instability)
- Severe confusion/agitation.

However, non-invasive BiPAP is sometimes used in drowsy or confused patients if it is decided that the patient is not suitable for tracheal intubation because of severe chronic lung disease.

Non-invasive BiPAP

Non-invasive ventilators have a simpler design compared with the ventilators on an ICU. This is because most were originally designed for home use. The

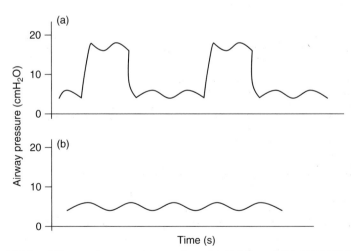

Figure 4.7 The difference between (a) non-invasive BiPAP and (b) CPAP. With non-invasive BiPAP, mechanical ventilation is superimposed on spontaneous breathing (see also Fig. 4.12).

disadvantage of this is that some are not adequately equipped in terms of monitoring and alarms when used in hospital.

The operator has to choose the appropriate type and size of mask and set basic ventilator controls: supplementary oxygen flow rate, IPAP, EPAP, backup respiratory rate (RR) and inspiratory time or inspiration to expiration (I:E) ratio.

Non-invasive BiPAP is used in certain patients with a mild-to-moderate acute respiratory acidosis (see Fig. 4.6). In an acute exacerbation of COPD, it is usual to begin with an IPAP of $15\,cmH_2O$ and an EPAP of $5\,cmH_2O$. The levels are then adjusted based on patient comfort, tidal volume achieved (if measured) and arterial blood gases.

The main indications for non-invasive BiPAP in the acute setting are:
• Exacerbation of COPD (pH low due to acute respiratory acidosis)
• Weaning from invasive ventilation.

There is a large body of evidence supporting non-invasive BiPAP in acute exacerbations of COPD (see Mini-tutorial: NIV for exacerbations of COPD). Non-invasive BiPAP can also be used as a step-down treatment in patients who have been intubated and ventilated on ICU. Weaning problems occur in at least 60% patients with COPD and this is a major cause of prolonged ICU stay. A randomised multi-centre trial has shown that non-invasive BiPAP is more successful in weaning than a conventional approach in patients with COPD [2]. Patients who failed a T-piece trial (breathing spontaneously with no support) 48 h after intubation were randomly assigned to receive either non-invasive BiPAP immediately after extubation or conventional weaning (a gradual reduction in ventilator support). The non-invasive BiPAP group took a shorter time to wean, had shorter ICU stays, a lower incidence of hospital-acquired pneumonia and increased 60-day survival. Other studies have reported similar findings.

Early trials of non-invasive BiPAP for pneumonia were discouraging, but a later prospective randomised trial of non-invasive BiPAP in community-acquired pneumonia (56 patients) showed a significant fall in RR and the need for intubation [3]. However, half of the patients in this study had COPD and it was carried out in an ICU. Previously well patients who require ventilation for pneumonia should be referred to an ICU as they are likely to need tracheal intubation.

Predictors of failure of non-invasive BiPAP in an acute exacerbation of COPD are:
• No improvement within 2 h
• High APACHE II score (Acute Physiological and Chronic Health Evaluation)
• Pneumonia
• Very underweight patient
• Neurological compromise
• pH <7.3 prior to starting NIV.

The updated UK guidelines on non-invasive BiPAP for exacerbations of COPD can be found on the British Thoracic Society website [4].

Mini-tutorial: NIV for exacerbations of COPD

An exacerbation of COPD requiring admission to hospital carries a 6–26% mortality [5]. One study found a 5-year survival of 45% after discharge and this reduced to 28% with further admissions [6]. Invasive ventilation for an exacerbation of COPD has an even higher mortality [7]. Ventilator-associated pneumonia is common and increases mortality still further. Non-invasive BiPAP is associated with less complications than tracheal intubation (see Fig. 4.8).

Most studies of non-invasive BiPAP in acute exacerbations of COPD have been performed in critical care areas. There have been at least half a dozen prospective randomised-controlled trials of non-invasive BiPAP vs standard care in acute exacerbations of COPD. The studies performed in ICUs showed a reduction in intubation rates and some also showed reduced mortality when compared to conventional medical therapy. None have directly compared non-invasive BiPAP with tracheal intubation. A multi-centre randomised-controlled trial of non-invasive BiPAP in general respiratory wards showed both a reduced need for intubation and reduced hospital mortality [8]. Patients with a pH below 7.3 on enrolment had a significantly higher failure rate and in-hospital mortality than those with an initial pH over 7.3, whether they received non-invasive BiPAP or not. It is therefore recommended that patients with a pH below 7.3 are monitored in a facility with ready access to tracheal intubation.

Non-invasive BiPAP should be commenced as soon as the pH falls below 7.35 because the further the degree of acidosis, the less the chances of improvement. It should be used as an adjunct to full medical therapy which treats the underlying cause of acute respiratory failure. In a 1-year prevalence study of nearly 1000 patients admitted with an exacerbation of COPD in one city, around 1 in 5 were acidotic on arrival in the Emergency Department, but 20% of these had a normal pH by the time they were admitted to a ward [9]. This included patients with an initial pH of <7.25, and suggests that non-invasive BiPAP should be commenced after medical therapy and controlled oxygen has been administered.

Patients on non-invasive BiPAP require close supervision because sudden deterioration can occur at any time. Simple measures, such as adjusting the mask to reduce excessive air leaks can make a difference to the success or otherwise of treatment. Basic vital signs frequently measured give an indication of whether or not non-invasive BiPAP is being effective. If non-invasive BiPAP does not improve respiratory acidosis in the first 2 h, tracheal intubation should be considered.

Non-invasive CPAP

Non-invasive CPAP was first introduced in the 1980s as a therapy for obstructive sleep apnoea (OSA). A tight-fitting face or nasal mask delivers a single positive pressure throughout the patient's respiratory cycle. In OSA, CPAP prevents pharyngeal collapse. CPAP can also be delivered through an endotracheal tube or tracheostomy tube in spontaneously breathing patients and is used this way during weaning from the ventilator.

The main indications for non-invasive CPAP in the acute setting are:

- To deliver increased oxygen in pneumonia or post-operative respiratory failure associated with atelectasis
- Acute cardiogenic pulmonary oedema.

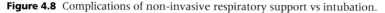

Non-invasive respiratory support	Tracheal intubation
Necrosis of skin over bridge of nose Aspiration Changes in cardiac output (less)	Pneumonia Barotrauma and volutrauma Changes in cardiac ouput Complications of sedation and paralysis Tracheal stenosis/tracheomalacia

Figure 4.8 Complications of non-invasive respiratory support vs intubation.

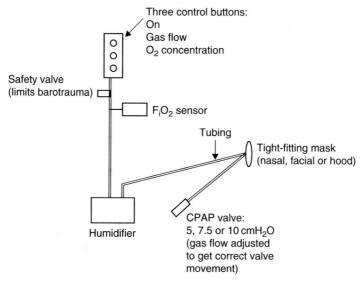

Figure 4.9 A CPAP circuit.

CPAP is employed in patients with acute respiratory failure to correct hypox-aemia. In the spontaneously breathing patient, the application of CPAP provides positive end-expiratory pressure (PEEP) that can reverse or prevent atelectasis, improve functional residual capacity and oxygenation. These improvements may prevent the need for tracheal intubation and can sometimes reduce the work of breathing. However, in patients with problems causing alveolar hypoventilation, mechanical ventilation rather than CPAP is more appropriate.

The inspiratory flow in a CPAP circuit needs to be high enough to match the patient's peak inspiratory flow rate. If this is not achieved, the patient will breathe against a closed valve with the risk that the generation of significant negative intrapleural pressure will lead to the development of pulmonary oedema. Look at the expiratory valve on a CPAP circuit in use. The valve should remain slightly open during inspiration (see Fig. 4.9).

Meta-analysis shows that non-invasive CPAP reduces the need for tracheal intubation in patients with acute cardiogenic pulmonary oedema (numbers needed to treat = 4) with a trend towards a reduction, but no significant dif-ference in mortality [10].

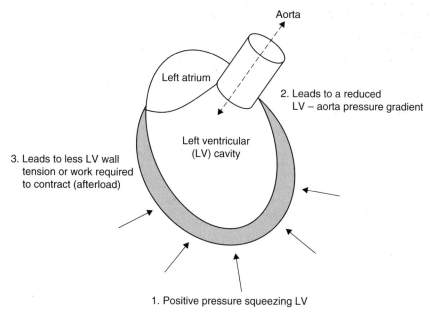

Figure 4.10 How CPAP reduces afterload in the failing heart.

In acute cardiogenic pulmonary oedema, CPAP 'squeezes' fluid out of the alveoli into the circulation. There is a decline in the level of shunt because of redistribution of lung water from the alveolar space to the perivascular cuffs. CPAP also has cardiovascular effects:

- Left ventricular function is improved because afterload is reduced (leading to an increase in stroke volume (SV)). This occurs because the increased intrathoracic pressure has a squeezing effect on the left ventricle. There is a subsequent reduction in the pressure gradient between the ventricle and the aorta which has the effect of reducing the work required during contraction (the definition of afterload) (see Fig. 4.10).
- Relief of respiratory distress leads to haemodynamic improvement and reversal of hypertension and tachycardia – probably through reduced sympathoadrenergic stimulation.

Non-invasive CPAP in acute cardiogenic pulmonary oedema is indicated when the patient has failed to respond to full medical therapy and there is an acute respiratory acidosis or hypoxaemia despite high-concentration oxygen therapy. However, patients who do not respond quickly to non-invasive CPAP should be referred for tracheal intubation.

Invasive respiratory support

In the past 'iron lungs' were used to apply an intermittent negative pressure to the thorax, thus inflating the lungs, but manual intermittent positive pressure

	Volume control	Pressure control
Delivery	Delivers a set tidal volume no matter what pressure this requires. This can cause excessively high peak pressures and barotrauma	If airway pressures are high, only small tidal volumes will be delivered. Not good if lung compliance keeps changing
Leaks	Poor compensation	Compensates for leaks well (e.g. poor fitting mask or circuit fault)
PEEP	Some flow/volume control ventilators cannot apply PEEP	PEEP easily added

Figure 4.11 Advantages and disadvantages of volume vs pressure control. PEEP: positive end-expiratory pressure.

ventilation (IPPV) was introduced during a large polio epidemic in Copenhagen in 1952. Mortality rates were lower than with previously used techniques. This heralded the introduction of ICUs.

ICU ventilators are set to deliver either a certain volume or a certain pressure when inflating the lungs. This is termed 'volume-control' or 'pressure-control' ventilation. These different modes of ventilation have their own advantages and disadvantages (see Fig. 4.11).

In volume-controlled ventilation, inhalation proceeds until a preset tidal volume is delivered and this is followed by passive exhalation. The set tidal volume is calculated from flow over a time period. A feature of this mode is that gas is often delivered at a constant inspiratory flow rate, resulting in peak pressures applied to the airways higher than that required for lung distension. Since the volume delivered is constant, airway pressures vary with changing pulmonary compliance and airway resistance. A major disadvantage is that excessive airway pressure may be generated, resulting in barotrauma, and so a pressure limit should be set by the operator.

In pressure-controlled ventilation a constant inspiratory pressure is applied and the pressure difference between the ventilator and lungs results in inflation until that pressure is attained. Passive exhalation follows. The volume delivered is dependent on pulmonary and thoracic compliance. A major advantage of pressure control is use of a decelerating inspiratory flow pattern, in which inspiratory flow tapers off as the lung inflates. This usually results in a more homogenous gas distribution throughout the lungs. A disadvantage is that dynamic changes in pulmonary mechanics may result in varying tidal volumes.

Sophisticated ventilators have been manufactured which incorporate the advantages of both modes and also interact with patients. ICU ventilators can switch between modes, so they can adapt to clinical circumstances and also facilitate weaning from the ventilator as the patient recovers. Ventilator modes are often described by what initiates the breath (trigger variable), what controls gas delivery during the breath (target or limit variable) and what terminates the breath (cycle variable). Hence, for example, BiPAP is machine or patient triggered, pressure targeted and time cycled.

The most commonly used ventilator modes on ICU are:
- BiPAP
- SIMV (synchronised intermittent mandatory ventilation)
- pressure support ventilation (PSV) also known as assisted spontaneous breaths (ASB)
- CPAP.

In the ICU setting, BiPAP is considered to be a single mode of ventilation that covers the entire spectrum of mechanical ventilation to spontaneous breathing. When the patient has no spontaneous breaths the ventilator acts as a pressure-controlled ventilator. When the patient has spontaneous breaths, the ventilator synchronises intermittently with the patient's breathing and spontaneous breaths can occur during any phase of the respiratory cycle without increasing airway pressure above the set maximum level, as can occur with conventional pressure-controlled ventilation (so-called 'fighting' the ventilator). When the patient is able to breathe more adequately, pressure support is used to augment every spontaneous breath.

The waveforms of these different ventilator modes are shown in Fig. 4.12.

The operator of an ICU ventilator can adjust the following main variables: F_iO_2, the inspiratory pressure, expiratory pressure (PEEP), backup RR, inspiratory time or I:E ratio and alarm limits (e.g. minimum and maximum tidal volumes).

PEEP

PEEP prevents the collapse of alveoli and this has several benefits:
- Improvement of V/Q matching
- Reduced lung injury from shear stresses caused by repeated opening and closing
- Prevention of surfactant breakdown in collapsing alveoli leading to improved lung compliance.

Lung disease is usually heterogeneous so recruitment of alveoli in one part of the lung may cause over-distension in another. PEEP also increases mean intrathoracic pressure which can reduce cardiac output (CO). PEEP is normally set to $5\,cmH_2O$ and increased if required. 'Best PEEP' for a particular patient can be elucidated from a ventilator's pressure–volume loop display.

The effects of mechanical ventilation

During IPPV there is reversal of the thoracic pump – the normal negative intrathoracic pressure during spontaneous inspiration which draws blood into the chest from the vena cavae, a significant aspect of venous return. With IPPV, venous return decreases during inspiration, and if PEEP is added venous return could be impeded throughout the respiratory cycle. This can cause hypotension. The degree of impairment of venous return is directly proportional to the mean intrathoracic pressure. So changes in ventilatory pattern, not just pressures, can cause cardiovascular changes.

At high lung volumes the heart may be directly compressed by lung expansion. This prevents adequate filling of the cardiac chambers. Ventricular

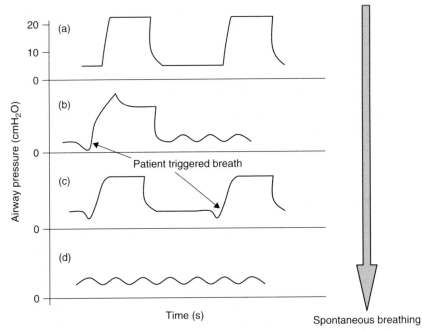

Figure 4.12 Waveforms of different ventilator modes. (a) BiPAP in a paralysed patient (i.e. no spontaneous breaths); (b) SIMV. There are spontaneous breaths between mechanical breaths. The ventilator synchronises mechanical breaths so that the lungs are not inflated during inspiration; (c) Augmented PSV (pressure support ventilation). The ventilator assists every spontaneous breath; (d) CPAP. Spontaneous ventilation plus a continuous positive airway pressure.

contractility is also affected. Elevated intrathoracic pressures directly reduce the left and right ventricular ejection pressure which is the difference between the pressure inside and outside the ventricular wall during systole. As a result, SV is reduced for a given end-diastolic volume.

IPPV can also reduce renal, hepatic and splanchnic blood flow.

These physiological changes during IPPV can be precipitously revealed when intubating critically ill patients. Marked hypotension and cardiovascular collapse can occur as a result of uncorrected volume depletion prior to tracheal intubation. This is compounded by the administration of anaesthetic drugs which cause vasodilatation and reduce circulating catecholamine levels as the patient losses consciousness.

The effects of mechanical ventilation are not as severe when the patient is awake and breathing spontaneously.

Although mechanical ventilation can be life saving for people with respiratory failure, poorly applied ventilation techniques can not only cause cardiovascular compromise but can also damage lung tissue and lead to ventilator-induced lung injury (VILI). In particular, large tidal volumes and extreme cyclical inflation and deflation have been shown to worsen outcome in acute lung injury (see Chapter 6).

Mini-tutorial: tracheal intubation in acute severe asthma

Tracheal intubation and ventilation can be a life-saving intervention. If indicated, it is important that it is performed sooner rather than later in acute severe asthma (when there is no response to maximum medical therapy). However, 10-min preparation beforehand is time well spent, particularly in those who are most unstable, as cardiovascular collapse can occur due to uncorrected volume depletion, the abolition of catecholamine responses and vasodilatation when anaesthetic drugs are given. Patients should be volume loaded prior to induction of anaesthesia and a vasopressor (e.g. ephedrine) kept ready to treat hypotension. Anaesthetic drugs are given cautiously to minimise any vasodilatory effect and drugs that cause histamine release are avoided if possible. In severe life-threatening asthma, maximum medical therapy might mean intravenous (i.v.) salbutamol, magnesium sulphate, hydrocortisone and nebulised or subcutaneous adrenaline [11]. Therapy should be started while preparations to intubate are underway. Following tracheal intubation, the patient is ventilated with a *long expiratory time* and this may mean only 6–8 breaths/min is possible. 'Permissive hypercapnia' is the term used when the $PaCO_2$ is allowed to rise in such situations, in order to prevent 'stacking'. This is when the next positive pressure is delivered before there has been enough time for expiration to occur (prolonged in severe lower airway obstruction). The lung volume slowly expands, reducing venous return and leading to a progressive fall in CO and BP. This is corrected by disconnecting the ventilator and allowing passive expiration to occur (which can take several seconds). The updated UK asthma guidelines can be found on the British Thoracic Society web site [12].

An algorithm outlining the management of respiratory failure is shown in Fig. 4.13.

Key points: respiratory failure

- Respiratory failure is characterised by a failure to ventilate or a failure to oxygenate or both.
- Treatment consists of oxygen therapy and treatment of the underlying cause.
- If there is no improvement, respiratory support is indicated and the type of respiratory support depends on the clinical situation.
- Respiratory support can be non-invasive (via a tight-fitting mask) or invasive (tracheal intubation).
- ICU ventilators utilise several different ventilator modes depending on the clinical situation.
- Invasive mechanical ventilation is associated with cardiovascular effects and VILI.

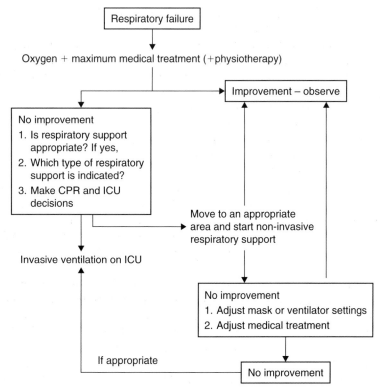

Figure 4.13 Algorithm for the management of respiratory failure. The appropriateness of any respiratory support should be decided by a senior doctor, for example, it would not be appropriated to ventilate a patient dying of terminal lung disease.

Self-assessment: case histories

1 A previously well 30-year-old woman is admitted in a coma from a drug overdose and responds only to painful stimuli. Arterial blood gases on air show: pH 7.24, $PaCO_2$ 8.32 kPa (64 mmHg), st bicarbonate 29 mmol/l, base excess (BE) +3, PaO_2 7.8 kPa (60 mmHg). The Emergency Department doctor diagnoses drug intoxication with aspiration pneumonia because of the hypoxaemia. What is your assessment?

2 Twenty-four hours later you are asked to assess the same patient for discharge as the hospital is in need of beds. She is alert and orientated, and her repeat arterial blood gases on air show: pH 7.6, $PaCO_2$ 3.1 kPa (24 mmHg), st bicarbonate 22 mmol/l, BE −3, PaO_2 9.1 kPa (70 mmHg). Should you discharge this patient?

3 A 24-year-old woman is admitted with acute severe asthma. Her vital signs are as follows: BP 100/60 mmHg, pulse 130/min, RR 40/min with poor respiratory effort, temperature 37°C and she is drowsy. Her arterial blood gases on 15 l/min oxygen via reservoir bag mask show: pH 7.15, $PaCO_2$

9.0 kPa (70 mmHg), st bicarbonate 22 mmol/l, BE −3, PaO_2 7 kPa (54 mmHg). What is your management?

4 Later on, in ICU the same patient develops hypotension (60/30 mmHg). The patient is sedated and paralysed, and the ventilator is set to 12 breaths/min. The inspiratory to expiratory ratio is 1:4, tidal volumes are 600 ml and peak airway pressures are 45 cmH_2O. What are the possible causes of the hypotension and what is your management?

5 A 50-year-old man is admitted with an exacerbation of his COPD. His arterial blood gases on a 28% Venturi mask show: pH 7.3, $PaCO_2$ 8.0 kPa (62 mmHg), st bicarbonate 29 mmol/l, BE +3, PaO_2 7 kPa (54 mmHg). What is your management?

6 A 40-year-old man with no past medical history is admitted with severe pneumonia. His vital signs are: BP 120/70 mmHg, pulse 110/min, RR 40/min, temperature 38°C and he is alert. His arterial blood gases on 15 l/min oxygen via reservoir bag mask show: pH 7.31, $PaCO_2$ 4.0 kPa (31 mmHg), PaO_2 6 kPa (46 mmHg), st bicarbonate 14 mmol/l, BE −7. What should you do?

7 You are called to see a 70-year-old man who is 2 days post-laparotomy. He has developed a cough with green sputum and a fever. His RR is increased (30/min) and his arterial blood gases on 10 l/min oxygen via Hudson mask show: pH 7.3, $PaCO_2$ 8.0 kPa (62 mmHg), st bicarbonate 29 mmol/l, BE +3, PaO_2 7.6 kPa (58 mmHg). What is your management?

8 A 60 kg 25-year-old woman with Guillain–Barré syndrome has been undergoing twice-daily forced vital capacity (FVC) measurements and treatment with i.v. immunoglobulin therapy. Her FVC has fallen below 1 l and her arterial blood gases on air now show: pH 7.3, $PaCO_2$ 7.5 kPa (58 mmHg), st bicarbonate 27 mmol/l, BE +2, PaO_2 10 kPa (77 mmHg). Her RR is 28/min. What do you do?

9 A 50-year-old woman is admitted with breathlessness. On examination she has a BP of 80 mmHg systolic which can only be measured by palpation. Her pulse is 110/min, RR 36/min and she is alert. Her chest sounds clear. The ECG shows sinus tachycardia with T-wave inversion in leads V_1–V_6 and her chest X-ray is normal. Arterial blood gases on 15 l/min oxygen via reservoir bag mask show: pH 7.25, $PaCO_2$ 3.0 kPa (23 mmHg), st bicarbonate 10 mmol/l, BE −12, PaO_2 12 kPa (92 mmHg). What is the diagnosis and what is your management?

10 A 70-year-old man with COPD is admitted *in extremis*. He has been more breathless for a few days. He responds to painful stimuli only, his BP is 130/60 mmHg, pulse 120/min and arterial blood gases on air show: pH 7.1, $PaCO_2$ 14.0 kPa (108 mmHg), st bicarbonate 20 mmol/l, BE −5, PaO_2 6 kPa (46 mmHg). What is your management?

Self-assessment: discussion

1 There is a low pH (acidaemia) due to a high $PaCO_2$ – a respiratory acidosis. The st bicarbonate is normal/high as expected. The PaO_2 is low. In this

situation, the PaO_2 could be low because of upper airway obstruction, aspiration pneumonia or hypoventilation caused by the drug overdose. The patient can be assessed clinically for signs of airway obstruction and the A-a gradient can be calculated to distinguish between a problem with gas exchange or hypoventilation. $PAO_2 = 0.21 \times 95 - 8.32/0.8 = 9.6\,kPa$. The A-a gradient is therefore $9.6 - 7.8 = 1.8\,kPa$ which is normal. This suggests hypoventilation rather than pneumonia is the cause of the low PaO_2. The management in this case still starts with ABC.

2 There is a high pH (alkalaemia) due to a low $PaCO_2$. The st bicarbonate is normal/low as expected. The PaO_2 has improved from before, but is still below the expected value. The A-a gradient can be calculated. $PAO_2 = 0.21 \times 95 - 3.1/0.8 = 16.1\,kPa$. The A-a gradient is therefore $16.1 - 9.1 = 7\,kPa$ which is abnormal. This could be explained by the development of aspiration pneumonia and requires further evaluation. The patient should not be discharged.

3 There is a low pH (acidaemia) due to a high $PaCO_2$ – a respiratory acidosis. The st bicarbonate is normal/high as expected. The PaO_2 is very low when compared with the F_iO_2 of approximately 0.8 (or 80%). Nine per cent of people with an attack of acute severe asthma have respiratory failure. One per cent patients with asthma have a fatal or near-fatal attack each year [11,12]. Previous life-threatening attacks increase the risk of death from asthma. You should have recognised, from the seriously abnormal vital signs, that this is a case of life-threatening asthma. Appropriate management therefore would be to call for help immediately, then assess and manage the airway, give the highest-concentration oxygen possible, assess and manage breathing (nebulised and/or i.v. bronchodilators and exclude pneumothorax), assess and manage circulation (give generous i.v. fluid – see Mini-tutorial: tracheal intubation in acute severe asthma) and move on to disability and examination once ABC are stable or help arrives. Unless there is a dramatic improvement, this patient requires the ICU team and tracheal intubation.

4 See the Mini-tutorial: tracheal intubation in acute severe asthma. However, apart from stacking, tension pneumothorax and hypovolaemia are other possible causes. Normally, ventilators are set so that peak airway pressures do not exceed 35–40 cmH$_2$O. This is slightly complicated by the fact that peak pressures in acute severe asthma do not necessarily reflect alveolar pressures but the ventilator pressures needed to overcome airway obstruction. PEEP is routinely added on ICU ventilators, but is not usually of benefit in acute severe asthma as patients already have significant intrinsic or auto-PEEP. In summary, an expert should supervise the ventilator requirements of any patient with acute severe asthma!

5 There is a low pH (acidaemia) due to a high $PaCO_2$ – a respiratory acidosis. The st bicarbonate is normal/high as expected. The PaO_2 is low. Apart from ABC, prompt medical management of his exacerbation of COPD may improve things. The oxygen could be increased to 35% and information about the patient's usual lung function sought. A chest X-ray should be

requested to exclude pneumothorax. If there is no prompt improvement of his respiratory acidosis with medical therapy, NIV should be started. Oxygen therapy is given through the ventilator mask, titrated to arterial blood gases. Intravenous fluid is often required for dehydration in breathless patients.

6 There is a low pH (acidaemia) due to a low st bicarbonate. The expected $PaCO_2$ should be lower, indicating a 'hidden' respiratory acidosis – he is tiring. This patient has serious abnormal vital signs and marked hypoxaemia despite a high concentration of oxygen. He may well be alert and talking, but he requires immediate assessment by the intensive care team. Generous fluid should be given for the metabolic acidosis, which is due to severe sepsis. Although some may be tempted to try non-invasive CPAP first, this will not alleviate respiratory fatigue and should not be performed outside an ICU in a situation like this. This patient is likely to require tracheal intubation soon.

7 There is a low pH (acidaemia) due to a high $PaCO_2$ – a respiratory acidosis. The st bicarbonate is normal/high as expected. The PaO_2 is low. Postoperative respiratory failure is caused by atelectasis due to a combination of recumbency, general anaesthesia and pain which prevents deep breathing and cough. Opioid analgesia also depresses respiration and cough. Retained secretions and even lobar collapse can occur. Management in this case should emphasise good pain relief (consider epidural analgesia) and urgent physiotherapy. The oxygen concentration should be increased and humidified. Antibiotics and sputum culture are required. If there is no improvement, the ICU team should be contacted. Non-invasive CPAP may be tried, but may not help when there is a significant problem with ventilation. Each patient is assessed on an individual basis.

8 There is a low pH (acidaemia) due to a high $PaCO_2$ – a respiratory acidosis. The st bicarbonate is normal and the PaO_2 is low. There is evidence of ventilatory failure (high $PaCO_2$ and increased RR) as a result of increasing respiratory muscle weakness (falling FVC). Closer examination may reveal a patient who is using accessory respiratory muscles and has a cough which is bovine in nature. Neurological examination may reveal poor bulbar function. Monitoring oxygen saturations and arterial blood gases in this condition are of little help in deciding when to institute respiratory support because abnormal arterial blood gases follow ventilatory failure rather than precede it. This is why the FVC is closely monitored. The usual cut-off is 15 ml/kg, below which tracheal intubation and ventilation are recommended. Up to one-third of patients with Guillain–Barré syndrome admitted to hospital require mechanical ventilation [13]. Autonomic neuropathy can accompany the syndrome, leading to tachycardia and hypotension which also require close observation especially during tracheal intubation which can precipitate asystole from profound vagal stimulation.

9 This patient is in shock. There is a low pH (acidaemia) due to a low st bicarbonate – a metabolic acidosis. The $PaCO_2$ is low as expected. The PaO_2 is also low compared with the F_iO_2. The A-a gradient is as follows: $PAO_2 = 0.8 \times 95 - 3.0/0.8 = 72.25$ kPa. A-a gradient $= 72.25 - 12 = 60.25$ kPa. What would cause such a significant problem with gas exchange, BP and the ECG changes with a normal chest X-ray? The answer is a massive pulmonary embolism. Treatment (after ABC) in this case includes i.v. thrombolysis which should be considered in pulmonary embolism causing shock and is as effective as surgical embolectomy. Recent literature suggests thrombolysis is safe and effective in 'sub-massive' pulmonary embolism as well [14].

10 There is a low pH (acidaemia) due to a high $PaCO_2$ – a respiratory acidosis. The st bicarbonate should be normal/high but it is low, indicating a 'hidden' metabolic acidosis as well, probably due to hypoperfusion (from dehydration). The PaO_2 is also low. His airway should be assessed and he requires oxygen to get his PaO_2 to around 8 kPa (60 mmHg). His breathing should be assessed next and medical therapy commenced. Non-invasive ventilation is usually contraindicated in patients with severe respiratory acidosis or who are unconscious. However, before proceeding to tracheal intubation, further information should be sought as to the severity of the patient's chronic lung disease. Has a discussion already taken place about tracheal intubation and ventilation between the patient and his specialist? Do the next of kin have information (e.g. an advanced directive) about what the patient would want in these circumstances? Sometimes, NIV is used as a 'second best' but more appropriate treatment. Each patient should be assessed individually by an experienced doctor.

References

1. Symonds AK (ed). *Non-invasive Respiratory Support*, Arnold Publishing, London, 2001.
2. Nava S, Ambrosino N, Clini E *et al.* Non-invasive mechanical ventilation in the weaning of patients with respiratory failure due to chronic obstructive pulmonary disease. A randomised controlled trial. *Annals of Internal Medicine* 1998; **128**: 721–728.
3. Confalonieri M, Potena A, Carbone G, Della Porta R, Tolley E and Meduri GU. Acute respiratory failure in patients with severe community-acquired pneumonia. A prospective randomised evaluation of non-invasive ventilation. *American Journal of Respiratory Critical Care Medicine* 1999; **160**: 1585–1591.
4. www.brit-thoracic.org.uk. Latest UK NIV guidelines for COPD.
5. Elliot MW. Non-invasive ventilation for exacerbations of chronic obstructive pulmonary disease. In: Symonds AK, ed. *Non-invasive Respiratory Support*. Arnold Publishing, London, 2001.
6. Vestbo J, Prescott E, Lange P, Schnohr P and Jenson G. Vital prognosis after hospitalisation for COPD: a study of a random population sample. *Respiratory Medicine* 1998; **92**: 772–776.
7. Hudson LD. Survival data in patients with acute and chronic lung disease requiring mechanical ventilation. *American Review of Respiratory Disease* 1989; **140**: S19–S24.
8. The YONIV Trial, Plant PK, Owen JL and Elliot MW. A multi-centre randomised controlled trial of the early use of non-invasive ventilation for acute exacerbations of

chronic obstructive pulmonary disease on general respiratory wards. *Lancet* 2000; **355(9219)**: 1931–1935.

9. Plant PK, Owen JL and Elliot MW. One year prevalence study of respiratory acidosis in acute exacerbations of COPD: implications for the provision of non-invasive ventilation and oxygen administration. *Thorax* 2000; **55**: 550–554.

10. Hughes CM. CPAP support reduces the need for intubation in patients with cardiogenic pulmonary oedema. *ACP J Club* 1999; **58**.

11. Wong B and Ball C. Asthma exacerbation. In: Ball C and Phillips R, eds. *Evidence-Based On-Call Acute Medicine*. Churchill Livingstone, London, 2001.

12. www.brit-thoracic.org.uk. Latest UK asthma guidelines.

13. Guillain–Barré syndrome. In: Yentis SM, Hirsch NP and Smith BG, eds. *Anaesthesia and Intensive Care A–Z*, 3rd edn. Butterworth Heinemann, London, 2004.

14. Konstantinides S *et al*. Heparin and alteplase compared with heparin alone in patients with submassive pulmonary embolism. *New England Journal of Medicine* 2002; **347(15)**: 1143–1150.

Further resource

• West JB. *Respiratory Physiology the Essentials,* 7th edn. Lippincott Williams and Wilkins, Philadelphia, 2005.

CHAPTER 5

Fluid balance and volume resuscitation

> **By the end of this chapter you will be able to:**
> - Understand the basic physiology of the circulation
> - Understand how normal fluid balance differs in illness
> - Assess the circulation
> - Understand the concept of a fluid challenge
> - Interpret central venous pressure readings
> - Know about the different types of fluid including blood
> - Apply this to your clinical practice

The previous chapters have concentrated on the airway (oxygen) and breathing in the acutely ill patients. This chapter is about the circulation and fluid balance. In acute illness, fluid therapy is needed to optimise oxygen delivery to the tissues.

Blood pressure

Blood pressure (BP) is determined by cardiac output (CO) and systemic vascular resistance (SVR):

$$BP = CO \times SVR$$

SVR may be thought of as the resistance against which the heart pumps. It is mainly determined by the diameter of arterioles, as small changes in their calibre produce large changes in resistance. Vasoconstriction raises BP and vasodilatation lowers BP. Various local factors affect SVR.

CO is determined by heart rate (HR) and stroke volume (SV):

$$CO = HR \times SV$$

CO falls below an HR of 40/min and above an HR of 140/min. SV is the amount of blood ejected with a single contraction and can also be described

---

Box 5.1 Factors that affect myocardial contractility

Increased contractility
- Sympathetic stimulation
- Positive inotropic drugs

Reduced contractility
- Parasympathetic stimulation
- Negatively inotropic drugs
- Ischaemia
- Hypoxaemia
- Acidosis
- Low calcium

Type of shock	CO	SVR
Cardiogenic	↓↓	↑
Hypovolaemic	↓	↑↑
Septic	↑↑	↓↓↓
Anaphylactic	↓	↓↓
Neurogenic	↓	↓↓↓

Figure 5.1 Characteristic haemodynamic variables in different types of shock. CO: cardiac output; SVR: systemic vascular resistance.

by the ejection fraction. It is defined as the difference between end-diastolic and end-systolic volume. SV is determined by three things: preload, contractility and afterload.

Preload is the initial length of a heart muscle fibre before contraction, as described in the Frank–Starling curve. In a normal heart, we take this to be the end-diastolic volume or the filling pressure of the left ventricle. In clinical practice, the central venous pressure (CVP) is used to estimate this, but with several limitations. Contractility is the amount of mechanical work that is done for a given preload and afterload. It is affected by various factors, as shown in Box 5.1. Afterload is defined as the tension developed in the ventricular wall during contraction, or how forcefully the ventricles have to contract to eject blood. It is affected by preload, SVR and positive pressure ventilation, which has a 'squeezing' effect on the ventricles.

Therefore, in order to optimise BP and perfusion of vital organs, all these factors need to be considered: HR, preload, contractility, afterload and SVR. These inter-relationships help to explain why different mechanisms cause shock, an inability to perfuse the tissues adequately. These inter-relationships are discussed further in Chapter 6 in the context of optimising oxygen delivery in severe sepsis. Fig. 5.1 illustrates the characteristic haemodynamic variables in different types of shock.

Fluid balance in health vs illness

Normally, people balance their daily fluid intake and output. A 70-kg adult has an approximate fluid intake of 1500 ml in liquid, 750 ml in food and 250 ml from metabolism. The approximate fluid output is 1500 ml in urine, 100 ml in faeces and 900 ml in insensible losses (e.g. sweating and breathing). If a healthy individual was 'nil by mouth', he would require maintenance fluid to maintain normal fluid balance and to replace insensible losses.

Maintenance fluid is calculated (in millilitre per hour) as follows:
- 4 ml/kg for the first 10 kg of the patient's weight
- 2 ml/kg for the second 10 kg of the patient's weight
- 1 ml/kg for every kg after that

So for the first 20 kg an adult requires 60 ml/h. A 70-kg adult would require 60 + 50 ml/h of fluid, roughly 2600 ml/day. Note that the fluid requirements of a 120-kg rugby player are totally different to the fluid requirements of an elderly 40-kg woman. Do not give everyone the proverbial '3 l/day'.

In addition, 50–150 mmol sodium and 20–40 mmol potassium is the average daily requirement for an adult. Hence an average water and electrolyte requirement can be found in 1l of 0.9% saline and 1.5l of 5% dextrose per day, plus some potassium.

However, *this applies to healthy people and many patients in hospital are physiologically stressed*. Illness alters fluid requirements, sodium homeostasis, how the body handles fluid and even the fluid compartments in the body. 'Maintenance fluid' as described above does not apply in these circumstances.

Fig. 5.2 illustrates water distribution in the body and the main fluid compartments. Human beings are 60% water, though this reduces with age. Two-thirds of this is intracellular water. Sodium and chloride provide the effective osmolality, or tonicity, of the extracellular compartment. The intracellular and extracellular spaces are separated by a semipermeable membrane which allows free movement of water. Plasma sodium and glucose changes result in movement of water across this membrane. Changes in osmolality are sensed by receptors that regulate the release of anti-diuretic hormone (ADH), which regulates water reabsorption by the kidneys.

Fluid requirements in illness

Many patients have increased fluid losses from:
- Fever (an extra 500 ml/day is required for every °C above 37)
- Breathlessness
- Diarrhoea/vomiting
- Haemorrhage
- Surgical drains
- Polyuria
- Third space losses (e.g. pancreatitis)
- Capillary leak in systemic inflammatory response syndrome (SIRS).

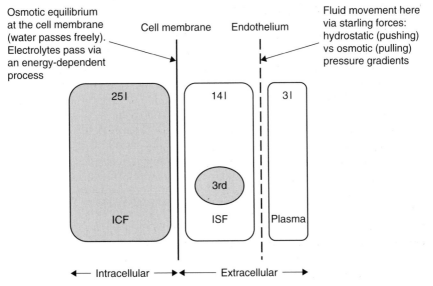

Figure 5.2 Water distribution in the body of a 70-kg man. ICF: intracellular fluid; ISF: interstitial fluid. Sodium changes in the extracellular compartments cause water shifts to and from cells, contracting or expanding the ICF. The third space is a non-exchangeable compartment in the ISF.

Some patients may need fluid, but require more careful monitoring for signs of fluid overload:
• Patients with heart failure
• Patients with significant *chronic* renal failure
• The elderly (because of reduced physiological reserve).

Sodium homeostasis in illness

Salt and water homeostasis is affected by physiological stress. ADH secretion increases due to a variety of stimuli: pain, opiate and anaesthetic drugs, surgery, mechanical ventilation and physiological stress. The elderly have impaired salt and water homeostasis, so iatrogenic disturbances in sodium are common in this group. In ill patients, where the serum sodium is below 140 (in the absence of sodium loss) one should assume that ADH is acting and avoid the administration of too much hypotonic fluid (5% dextrose or dextrose 4% saline 0.18%), which could precipitate hyponatraemia. Potassium is also commonly affected by illness as well as long-term medication, so it is added to a fluid regime after the blood results are known.

The commonly used fluids available in the UK for volume resuscitation (0.9% saline and gelatines) contain sodium. This results in critically ill patients being given significant amounts of sodium. In trauma, surgery, bleeding or severe sepsis, the body already avidly retains sodium (via the

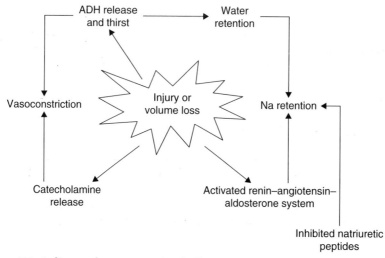

Figure 5.3 Sodium and water retention in illness.

renin–angiotensin–aldosterone axis) and water (via ADH), as illustrated in Fig. 5.3 and this tends to reduce urine output; 0.9% saline also contains significant amounts of chloride which causes a mild hyperchloraemic metabolic acidosis, renal vasoconstriction and oliguria.

Critically ill patients have reduced renal concentrating ability and need to excrete more water to get rid of their solute load. Typically, a recovering patient will excrete this sodium and water load over the next 2–5 days. But if there are further complications (e.g. infection or prolonged inflammation), a vicious circle ensues in which ever increasing amounts of sodium and chloride exacerbate oedema and tissue hypoperfusion [1]. Although sodium and chloride loading is unavoidable in volume resuscitation, it can be limited by using colloids and crystalloids together, as colloids contain less sodium per volume expansion effect. This is common practice in the UK.

How the body handles fluid in illness

Water-depleted (dehydrated) or volume-depleted patients retain fluid in the intravascular compartment for longer, whereas patients with capillary leak retain fluid in the intravascular compartment for a shorter time. Capillary leak occurs as part of the inflammatory response to a range of insults. It occurs within minutes of injury and is proportional to the severity of the insult. Holes literally appear in the endothelium, and protein and water leaks out into the interstitial space, causing oedema and impaired oxygen delivery to the tissues. An uncontrolled response is seen in SIRS, as shown in Fig. 5.4. A typical patient with SIRS (e.g. severe acute pancreatitis) has peripheral oedema and bilateral basal crackles in the lungs, with intravascular volume depletion.

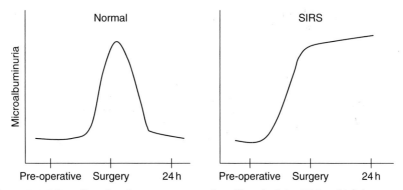

Figure 5.4 Microalbuminuria as a measure of capillary leak in SIRS, which is an exaggerated, uncontrolled inflammatory response to a range of insults including major surgery, trauma, burns, pancreatitis or infection. The normal response is shown on the left.

The concept of the third space

Fluid can accumulate in non-functioning spaces such as the peritoneum, pleura or bowel. The concept of the third space was developed to explain the phenomenon that some post-operative patients require more replacement fluid than their measurable losses. Third space losses are seen in pancreatitis, bowel obstruction and after laparotomy. See Mini-tutorial: fluid balance in alcoholic liver disease with ascites.

To summarise, one should aim to give fluid for a reason:
- For maintenance: Hartmann's (or 0.9% saline and 5% dextrose in combination)
- For water loss: 5% dextrose
- For volume expansion: blood or colloid and 0.9% saline (see Mini-tutorial: the crystalloid vs colloid debate)
- For nutrition: food and water via nasogastric tube.

When prescribing fluid, consider the weight of the patient and maintenance requirements, then consider any changes in fluid requirements which will have occurred due to illness. Then think what the fluid is for and choose accordingly. See case histories for examples.

Assessing volume status

Sometimes it is easy to see that a patient is hypovolaemic and requires i.v. fluid. Other times it is easy to see that a patient is fluid overloaded. But in many cases patients do not fit easily into either category. There are also many complex situations in which patients develop oedema but still require i.v. fluid (e.g. SIRS). The following are used to determine a patient's intra-vascular volume status:
- History
- Bedside examination

Mini-tutorial: fluid balance in alcoholic liver disease with ascites

Fluid balance in patients with cirrhosis and ascites can be difficult because of the changes in sodium and fluid compartments which occur. There is increased total body water and sodium, but reduced intravascular volume is caused by:
- Poor oral intake
- Gastrointestinal bleeding
- Sepsis
- Splanchnic vasodilatation
- Low CO relative to the dilated arterial bed.

Patients typically have a low urea (impaired hepatic function) and creatinine (less muscle mass). Hyponatraemia is common, caused by ADH stimulation (see Fig. 5.3). In acutely ill patients with decompensated liver disease, the key considerations in fluid balance are:
- Early nasogastric feeding, which improves outcome [2] and reduces the need for maintenance fluid.
- Restoration of intravascular volume, if there is sepsis or worsening renal function. The administration of human albumin solution (HAS) in these situations improves outcome [3,4], although it is likely that it is the restoration of intravascular volume rather than the particular fluid used which has this effect.
- Blood transfusion if the patient is bleeding.
- Avoiding excess 5% dextrose infusions which may precipitate hyponatraemia and central pontine myelinolysis.

A rising creatinine, even if still within the normal range, is significant in cirrhosis and may herald the development of hepatorenal syndrome. This is renal failure associated with cirrhosis and not due to sepsis, bleeding or nephrotoxic drugs. Treatment is:
- To relieve increased intra-abdominal pressure caused by tense ascites which can compromise the renal circulation.
- Restore intravascular volume using colloids (less sodium per volume expansion effect) and some crystalloids (0.9% saline).
- Administer a vasopressor (e.g. Terlipressin), which reverses the extreme splanchnic arterial vasodilatation seen in these patients, effectively increasing arterial blood volume.

These patients should be cared for by a specialist team.

- Response to fluid challenges
- CVP readings.

History alone can point to hypovolaemia. A patient may have been admitted with bowel obstruction and vomiting, bleeding, sepsis or not eating and drinking.

Simple bedside observations are vitally important in the evaluation of volume status and are also used to monitor the effectiveness of fluid resuscitation. As a patient becomes more and more volume depleted, certain compensatory responses occur which can be identified. BP falls late. In haemorrhage, the patient

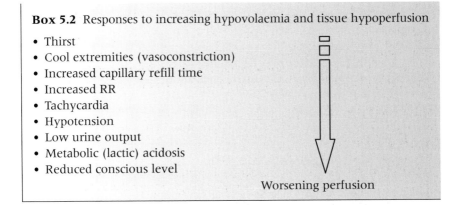

Box 5.2 Responses to increasing hypovolaemia and tissue hypoperfusion

- Thirst
- Cool extremities (vasoconstriction)
- Increased capillary refill time
- Increased RR
- Tachycardia
- Hypotension
- Low urine output
- Metabolic (lactic) acidosis
- Reduced conscious level

Worsening perfusion

has already lost 30% of circulating volume by the time hypotension occurs. The responses to increasing hypovolaemia and tissue hypoperfusion are summarised in Box 5.2. The bedside examination must take into account the *overall picture*, as no sign is reliable in isolation and some signs will not be present at all.

Thirst

Thirst can be a useful clinical finding when combined with other markers of hypovolaemia. However, dry oxygen therapy and 'nil by mouth' status may also contribute to the sensation of thirst. The elderly have an impaired thirst mechanism.

Cool extremities

Cool extremities can be a sign of hypovolaemia, as it reflects compensatory vaso-constriction. A young patient who is bleeding will appear pale and clammy because of sympathetic activation and thus have a normal BP. A capillary refill time of more than 2 s is abnormal. In sepsis, cool extremities may not occur due to pathological vasodilatation. Nevertheless, cool extremities in combination with a metabolic (lactic) acidosis has been found to be a reliable marker of hypoperfusion [5].

Increased respiratory rate

Respiratory rate (RR) increases in hypovolaemia as the body tries to compensate by increasing oxygen delivery and the removal of acid-waste products. An increased RR can be an early marker of acidosis and a rate of above 20 breaths/min is abnormal. RR is infrequently monitored in hospital and its significance can be missed. Patients may have an increased RR for other reasons, such as lung disease or pain.

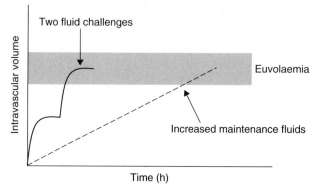

Figure 5.5 The effect of fluid challenges vs maintenance fluids on intravascular volume.

Tachycardia

Tachycardia (HR >90/min) occurs in hypovolaemia. However, certain patients may not get a tachycardia: the elderly, athletes, some patients with pacemakers and those on rate-slowing medication (e.g. beta-blockers).

Hypotension and low urine output

Hypotension and low urine output are late signs in volume depletion. A normal BP can be falsely reassuring – if a patient is normally hypertensive, a relatively normal BP can cause hypoperfusion and impaired renal function (see Chapter 7).

Metabolic (lactic) acidosis

The amount of lactate produced by the tissues during anaerobic metabolism correlates with the degree of tissue hypoperfusion. Serial arterial blood gas measurements can be helpful to assess the adequacy of resuscitation. Lactate is discussed further in Chapter 6 in the context of resuscitation in severe sepsis.

Response to fluid challenges

If there is any uncertainty about a patient's volume status, a fluid challenge is a safe and simple way to assess this further. The aim of a fluid challenge is to produce a small but rapid increase in intravascular volume and then to assess the response by a repeated bedside examination. Simply increasing maintenance fluids is not an effective way to treat or assess possible hypovolaemia. As Fig. 5.5 shows, increasing maintenance fluids takes a longer time to restore intravascular volume. Hypoperfusion, if present, needs to be treated as quickly as possible. A fluid challenge should be given through a large bore cannula

Size of cannula	Colour code	Flow rate (millilitre per minute)
24G	Yellow	18
22G	Blue	36
20G	Pink	61
18G	Green	90
16G	Grey	200
14G	Brown	300

Figure 5.6 Flow rates of different sized venous cannulae. The Hagen–Poiseuille equation states that flow is proportional to the pressure gradient and radius (to the power of four) of a tube and inversely proportional to the fluid viscosity and length of the tube. The relatively small diameter and long length of a central line makes it less suitable for resuscitation when fluid needs to be given quickly.

(14–16G) and a wide diameter giving set so that it can be given quickly. Fig. 5.6 shows the flow rates of different sized venous cannulae.

The quantity of fluid in a fluid challenge varies according to the situation. In trauma and sepsis these have been defined in international guidelines [6,7]. In a situation where the patient is stable and you wish to assess volume status, a fluid challenge is 500 ml 0.9% saline or 250-ml colloid, such as a gelatine or 6% hydroxyethyl starch (HES) *over 5 min*. Repeated or larger boluses are given in the treatment of hypovolaemia. The different types of fluid are discussed later. The reason why a fluid challenge is given over 5 min is because most fluids stay in the circulation for only a short time, less than an hour in the case of crystalloids and only a few hours in the case of commonly used colloids. Giving a fluid challenge over 1 h would have the same effect as running a bath with the plug pulled out.

How much fluid is enough? It is often difficult to know when a patient is euvolaemic using only the bedside assessment. As a rule, another fluid challenge is safe if the lungs are clear. If signs of fluid overload develop (increasing crackles in the lungs and interstitial shadowing on the chest X-ray), or the patient is requiring large amounts of fluid, more sophisticated monitoring and possibly other treatments are required (e.g. vasopressors/inotropes or haemorrhage control).

CVP readings
Central venous cannulation is used for the following:
- Delivering irritant or vaso-active drugs
- Central venous pressure (CVP) measurements
- As a conduit (e.g. pacing wires)
- Venous access.

The CVP is expressed in mmHg when transduced, that is attached directly to a monitor when the mean value is taken, or cmH_2O when measured manually using a manometer when the end-expiratory value is taken. 10 mmHg is equivalent to 13 cmH_2O. The CVP can be used to estimate a patient's volume status, especially if the bedside assessment is difficult. It is used as an estimate of left ventricular filling pressure or preload. In a healthy person, this estimate holds true. However, there are many other factors which affect the CVP.

CVP is reduced by hypovolaemia or vasodilatation, both of which require fluid. However, the CVP can increase for a number of reasons:
- Vasoconstriction
- Right heart failure (e.g. posterior myocardial infarction)
- Tricuspid regurgitation
- Constrictive pericarditis or tamponade
- Raised intrathoracic pressure (e.g. mechanical ventilation)
- Pneumothorax
- Lung diseases with pulmonary hypertension (e.g. chronic obstructive pulmonary disease (COPD), acute respiratory distress syndrome (ARDS))
- Fluid overload.

If a healthy person started to bleed, the CVP would initially rise due to compensatory vasoconstriction. It would fall back to normal as a result of fluid administration. This is the opposite of what most junior doctors think when asked about the CVP. The most important concept is that the CVP is a pressure, and not a volume. Many things affect the pressure in the right heart that have nothing to do with volume: valve disease, lung disease (afterload), vascular tone (preload) and muscle compliance. So although the CVP is being used as an estimate of left ventricular preload, it has several limitations.

Single CVP readings are irrelevant. The bedside assessment *and the response of the CVP to a fluid challenge* are what is used to assess volume status. It is possible to have a normal or even high CVP reading and be volume depleted. Therefore, there is no 'normal' CVP value, although a CVP below 10 mmHg is considered low and generally requires fluid.

Fig. 5.7 illustrates how the CVP is interpreted using the response to fluid challenges. If the CVP remains unchanged, or rises but then quickly falls back to the original value, the patient requires more fluid. If the CVP rises to above 10 mmHg and stays there, the patient is probably adequately filled. If the first CVP reading is above 10 mmHg, and the patient is not fluid overloaded according to the bedside assessment, give a fluid challenge to assess the response. The patient is adequately filled when the CVP 'goes up and stays up'.

Some patients continue to show signs of inadequate perfusion (cool extremities, increased RR, tachycardia, hypotension, oliguria and metabolic acidosis) even though they have an optimal intravascular volume, for example in cardiogenic shock and sepsis. More advanced monitoring and treatment with vaso-active drugs is required. Vasopressors and inotropes are discussed in Chapter 6.

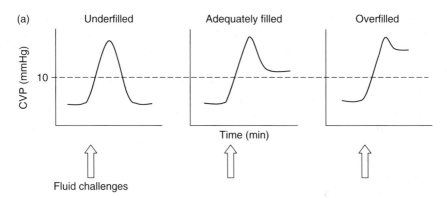

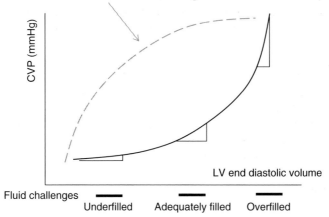

Figure 5.7 (a) The response of the CVP to fluid challenges. (b) In a hypovolaemic patient, an increase in SV with no significant rise in CVP would be expected. In the overfilled patient, a rise in CVP with no significant rise in SV would be expected.

Other ways to monitor the circulation

Pulmonary artery (PA) or Swan–Ganz catheters are used in an attempt to measure left heart pressures more directly than the CVP catheter, but there are still several limitations. PA catheters can also be used to estimate CO and SVR. There is no evidence that using a PA catheter improves outcome [8] and a number of less invasive techniques have been developed. Current practice in the UK is to use a PA catheter in certain intensive care unit (ICU) situations if the risk:benefit ratio to the patient has been considered, it is inserted by a properly trained individual and the measurements gained are used in context, taking into account the history and bedside examination. Further information on the PA catheter can be found in the Appendix on practical procedures.

Oesophageal Doppler, arterial waveform analysis and modified Fick techniques are examples of less invasive haemodynamic monitoring techniques. Oesophageal Doppler can estimate CO by measuring the velocity of blood flow (V_f) and the cross-sectional area of the aorta (CSA_a) via a probe placed through the nose. At the level between the 5th and 6th thoracic vertebrae the aorta is adjacent and parallel to the oesophagus. Aortic blood flow = $V_f \times CSA_a$. The probe measures blood flow in the descending aorta, which is typically 70% of CO, allowing for blood flow to the aortic arch branches. In this way, SV and CO can be estimated. If the BP is known, SVR can also be derived. As with all haemodynamic monitoring techniques, there are limitations, but oesophageal Doppler has been shown to be comparable to PA catheterisation.

The PiCCO system uses a central venous catheter and a thermistor-tipped femoral arterial line. The arterial line allows pulse contour analysis, and a thermodilution technique allows estimation of intrathoracic blood volume. A known volume of cold saline is rapidly injected into the central venous cannula. A temperature difference is detected by the femoral thermistor and a dissipation curve is generated. From this and other data, CO, SV and SVR can be derived. This system is also reported to have similar accuracy to PA catheterisation.

The LiDCO system is similar, but uses a small bolus of lithium chloride rather than cold saline.

All of these systems make assumptions in the same way that the CVP does, and rely on derived data. Trends are more important than single readings and data must take into account the bedside assessment in order to be interpreted correctly. A danger with sophisticated monitoring is the reliance on numbers rather than clinical assessment, which could lead to inappropriate management decisions.

Different types of fluid

The terms crystalloid and colloid were coined in the 19th century by Thomas Graham, who distinguished materials in aqueous solution which would or would not pass through a parchment membrane. The word crystalloid refers to crystalline substances like salt and the word colloid comes from the Greek word for glue.

Crystalloids

Crystalloids are substances which form a true solution and pass freely through semipermeable membranes. They contain water, dextrose and electrolytes, and stay in the intravascular compartment for about 45 min.

Crystalloids pass easily through capillary and glomerular membranes, but although they do not diffuse through cell membranes, membrane pumps and metabolism soon alter their distribution. Their composition varies depending on the type of solution. Sodium is the particle responsible for plasma volume expansion and this determines the initial distribution of a crystalloid; 5%

dextrose is basically free water as it does not contain sodium and distributes to both the intracellular fluid and extracellular fluid. It cannot be used in volume resuscitation.

Crystalloids are used to restore extracellular electrolyte and volume deficits. They are cheap, safe and readily available. The only limitation of crystalloids is the amount of fluid needed to effectively expand intravascular volume; 3–4 l of crystalloid are required to replace 1 l of blood, because only one-fourth of the volume reaches the circulation. There are theoretical disadvantages to this. Oedema occurs more commonly when crystalloids are used in resuscitation. The most commonly used crystalloids are:

- 0.9% sodium chloride
- 5% dextrose
- dextrose 4% saline 0.18%
- Hartmann's solution.

When 0.9% sodium chloride is given to healthy volunteers they develop nausea, abdominal cramps and a hyperchloraemic metabolic acidosis (with a normal anion gap) [9].

Hartmann's solution more closely resembles the extracellular fluid and contains lactate which is metabolised to bicarbonate, mainly in the liver, over 1–2 h. Lactated Ringer's solution is the same thing used in the USA. Hartmann's is preferred for maintenance fluid because its constituents closely match that of plasma. It is also used in volume resuscitation. It is avoided in certain patients: renal failure because of the risk of hyperkalaemia (though the actual risk is small) and liver failure because of the risk of lactic acidosis. Some of the lactate is metabolised to glucose and this has to be borne in mind for patients with diabetes. The calcium content of Hartmann's means that it may form clots if mixed with stored blood (which contains citrate) in the same i.v. line. Fig. 5.8 shows the electrolyte content of common crystalloids.

	Na^{2+}	K^+	Ca^{2+}	Cl^-	HCO_3	Osmolality	pH	Other
Plasma	140	4	2.3 (9.2)	100	26	285–295	7.0	
Sodium chloride 0.9%	154	0	0	154	0	308	5.0	
Dextrose 5%	0	0	0	0	0	252	4.0	Dextrose 50 g/l
Dextrose 4% saline 0.18%	30	0	0	0	30	255	4.0	Dextrose 40 g/l
Hartmann's	131	5	2 (8)	111	0	278	6.5	29 lactate
Sodium bicarbonate 8.4%	1000	0	0	0	1000	2000	8	

Figure 5.8 Electrolyte content of common crystalloids in mmol/l (mg/dl).

Colloids

Colloids are substances that do not form true solutions and do not pass through semipermeable membranes. They remain confined to the intravascular compartment, at least initially. Some are 'plasma expanders', because they have a higher osmolality than plasma and draw water from the interstitial space.

Different colloids have very different properties. The most commonly used colloids are:

- *Gelatines (e.g. Gelofusine and Haemaccel)*: Gelatine is a degradation product of animal collagen and is inexpensive and readily available. Different brands vary in electrolyte content. The calcium content of Haemaccel means that it may form clots if mixed with stored blood (which contains citrate) in the same i.v. line.
- *Hydroxyethylated starch (HES)*: This is derived from amylopectin, a plant polymer and contains no electrolytes. Unmodified starch is unsuitable as a plasma substitute since it is broken down rapidly by amylase. The hydroxyethylation of starch protects the polymer against breakdown. Different products with different mean molecular weights exist. Larger particles have a higher degree of protection from metabolism and give a more prolonged effect. HES is used with crystalloids in patients with capillary leak. It cannot constitute more than 30% of volume replacement, otherwise an osmotic nephrosis and renal failure can occur.
- *Human albumin solution (HAS)*: Albumin is the fraction of plasma which provides the main part of the circulation's osmotic pressure and has therefore been used as a plasma substitute. It is derived from human plasma and is heat sterilised, so it is virtually disease free; 4.5% HAS reflects normal plasma; 20% HAS has water and salt removed. HAS was mainly used to replace fluid losses in burns where albumin loss was also a problem, but see Mini-tutorial: controversies over albumin. The major limitations to the use of HAS are high production costs and limited supplies.

The molecular weight determines the retention time and duration of colloidal effect in the circulation. Lower-molecular-weight particles have a higher osmotic effect, but are rapidly excreted by the kidneys in contrast to larger particles. Allergic reactions can occur with colloid infusions. Colloids can also affect coagulation through various mechanisms, but with modern colloids

Mini-tutorial: controversies over albumin

In 1998 a meta-analysis by the Cochrane Injuries Group Albumin Reviewers questioned the practice of many doctors in ICUs [10]. Using data from 24 studies involving 1419 patients, the meta-analysis reported that the administration of albumin to critically ill patients increased the absolute risk of death by 6%, suggesting one extra death for every 17 patients given albumin. The authors recommended that albumin should not be administered to critically ill patients outside rigorously conducted randomised trials. The validity of the studies included in the systematic review was extensively debated. A later publication pointed out that more than half the trials included studies which did not reflect current practice.

The Saline vs Albumin Evaluation (SAFE) [11] study was initiated to address this uncertainty. 6997 patients admitted to ICUs were randomised to receive either 4% albumin or 0.9% saline. No significant difference in mortality, length of stay in ICU or hospital was seen in the albumin and saline groups. The investigators concluded that albumin and saline could be considered clinically equivalent treatments for intravascular volume resuscitation in a heterogeneous ICU population. However, it was postulated that further analysis on different subsets of patients may show differences.

Albumin is sometimes given to treat hypoalbuminaemia, which occurs in critical illness. This has not been shown to improve outcome when compared with synthetic colloids. Albumin leaks from the circulation in critical illness, but serum albumin levels do not correlate with the osmotic pressure of the intravascular compartment. Studies have shown similar osmotic pressures in critically ill patients with low vs normal albumins.

used in combination with crystalloids this is rarely associated with clinical bleeding. Fig. 5.9 shows the electrolyte content of common colloids.

Blood

The following are indications for blood transfusion:
- To restore intravascular volume in haemorrhage
- To restore oxygen carrying capacity.

Giving blood carries a small risk and uses a valuable resource. Apart from in haemorrhage, or before major surgery, blood transfusion is generally not indicated until the haemoglobin is less than 8.0 g/dl.

Stored whole blood has a haematocrit of 40% but plasma, platelets and other components are removed, leaving concentrated red cells with a haematocrit of 60%. It can be stored at 1–6°C for 28 days. Acid citrate dextrose is one of the most common additives used to prevent clotting. The acid acts as a

	Na^{2+}	K^+	Ca^{2+}	Cl^-	Osmolality	pH	Duration of volume effect
Plasma	140	4	2.3 (9.2)	100	285–295	7.0	
Gelofusine	154	0.4	0.4 (1.6)	120	274	7.4	2–3 h
Haemaccel	145	5.1	6.25 (25)	145	301	7.3	2–3 h
Albumin 4.5%	145	<2	0	145	290	7.4	6–12 h
Albumin 20%	145	<2	0	145	290	7.4	6–12 h
*HES 6%	154	0	0	154	310	5.5	7–24 h

Figure 5.9 Electrolyte content of common colloids in mmol/l (mg/dl). *Also contains 60 g starch.

Box 5.3 Complications of blood transfusion

Immunological
- Haemolysis
- Anaphylaxis

Infective
- Rarely, red cells can become contaminated with bacteria during storage. There is rapid development of severe sepsis
- In UK blood is screened for hepatitis B and C, HIV and syphilis. Donors undergo rigorous screening with several exclusion criteria. Since 1998, 95% of white cells are removed because of the theoretical risk of new variant Creutzfeldt–Jakob disease (nvCJD) transmission
- Other infections may be transmitted (e.g. cytomegalovirus)

Massive blood transfusion (e.g. 10 units within 6 h) has particular problems:
- Thrombocytopaenia
- Coagulopathy
- Hypothermia
- Hypocalcaemia
- Hyperkalaemia
- Metabolic acidosis followed by metabolic alkalosis due to citrate (which metabolises to bicarbonate)
- Acute respiratory distress syndrome (ARDS)
- Impaired oxygen delivery (left shift of O_2 dissociation curve in stored blood for 24 h)

buffer, the citrate binds calcium which inhibits clotting, and the dextrose acts as a substrate for red cells. Working platelets are reduced to virtually zero after 24 h of storage and clotting factors V and VIII are reduced to 50% after 21 days.

In serious haemorrhage, there are different types of blood matching available:
- O-negative blood is immediately available
- Type-specific blood (group and rhesus state only) is ready in 10 min
- Fully cross-matched blood is available in 30 min .

The risks of transfusion decrease with more specific matching. Transfusion reactions are rare but can occur with only small amounts of blood and death occurs in 1 in 100,000 transfusions. Complications of blood transfusion are shown in Box 5.3. Fluid overload can also occur.

The TRICC study [12] was a large randomised prospective trial which looked at blood transfusions on ICU. The first group (418 patients) was randomised to a restrictive policy in which blood transfusion was triggered at a haemoglobin of 7 g/dl and maintained at 7–9. The second group (420 patients) was randomised to receive blood if the haemoglobin fell below 10 g/dl and was maintained at 10–12. There was no advantage for patients with higher haemoglobins overall and blood transfusions were reduced by 54%. However, in less severely ill patients under the age of 55 years, outcome was improved in the restricted transfusion group. An association between increased mortality and number of transfusions was also found in the ABC and CRIT study [13,14]. Current practice is to restrict blood transfusion based on these studies. Patients with coronary artery disease and the elderly may require special consideration, and research is ongoing in this area.

Mini-tutorial: the crystalloid vs colloid debate

Despite much debate concerning the choice of fluid in volume resuscitation, the crystalloid vs colloid debate continues unabated.

Crystalloids resuscitate the intravascular and interstitial compartments. They are quickly redistributed and large volumes are therefore required to expand intravascular volume. This causes problems with interstitial oedema, which has theoretical disadvantages (impaired gas exchange and wound healing). Colloids expand intravascular volume more quickly, with less sodium and chloride loading. However, colloids are more expensive and allergic reactions can occur.

All crystalloids and most colloids used to expand intravascular volume contain saline. The mild metabolic acidosis that occurs can be misinterpreted as a sign of under resuscitation, although hyperchloraemic acidosis has a normal anion gap.

Extensive research has failed to show the superiority of colloids or crystalloids in the resuscitation of acutely ill patients. A recent Cochrane Systematic Review [15] concluded that there was no evidence of benefit of colloids over crystalloids and the expense of colloids raises questions about their use. But all colloids are not the same and this is the problem with meta-analyses. There are theoretical reasons why certain subgroups of patients may benefit from colloids as well as crystalloids. Patients are never resuscitated using only colloids. Research has yet to answer these questions.

Key points: fluid balance and volume resuscitation

- Understanding the physiology of the circulation is important in the assessment and treatment of patients.
- Illness alters fluid requirements, sodium homeostasis, how the body handles fluid and even the fluid compartments in the body.
- Simple bedside observations are vitally important in the evaluation of volume status.
- Fluid challenges are used to assess the circulation or treat hypovolaemia.
- Any form of haemodynamic monitoring must be interpreted in clinical context and trends are more important than single readings.
- There are many different types of fluid available – think why the fluid is needed and give fluid for a reason.

Self-assessment: case histories

1 An 85-year-old man is admitted with 'general deterioration' for 2–3 days, not eating or drinking and is hypotensive. He has a long-term urinary catheter inserted for obstruction. On examination he is drowsy, pulse is 70/min, BP 80/50 mmHg, RR 24/min, SpO_2 94% on air and temperature 34°C. His hands and feet are cool to touch. His blood results show: Na 155 mmol/l, K 4.0 mmol/l, urea 36 mmol/l (blood urea nitrogen (BUN) 100 mg/dl) and creatinine 260 μmol/l (3.12g/dl). He weighs 60 kg. What is your management?

2 A 40-year-old man with alcoholic liver disease is admitted generally unwell with abdominal swelling. On examination he appears malnourished and has a large amount of ascites. He is jaundiced. His vital signs are: alert, pulse 90/min, BP 90/60 mmHg, RR 18/min, SpO_2 95% on air, temperature 38°C. His blood results show: Na 125 mmol/l, K 3.4 mmol/l, urea 10 mmol/l (BUN 27.7 mg/dl), creatinine 100 μmol/l (1.2 mg/dl) and haemoglobin 14 g/dl. He weighs 50 kg. What is your management?

3 A 60-year-old man returns to the ward, following a laparotomy for bowel obstruction. You are informed that his urine output for the last 2 h has been less than 30 ml/h. He weighs 70 kg. In theatre he received 2 l of Hartmann's, 2 units of blood and 500 ml Gelofusine. His vital signs are: alert, pulse 80/min, BP 140/70 mmHg, RR 20/min, SpO_2 98% on 2 l oxygen via nasal cannulae and temperature 37.5°C. What is your management?

4 A 55-year-old man is on the coronary care unit following an infero-lateral myocardial infarction when he develops a low urine output. His vital signs are: alert, pulse 90/min, BP 100/50 mmHg, RR 22/min, SpO_2 98% on 2 l oxygen via nasal cannulae and temperature 37°C. His lungs are clear. He has cool hands and feet. His arterial blood gases show: pH 7.34, $PaCO_2$ 4.0 kPa (27 mmHg), st bicarbonate 17 mmol/l, base excess (BE) −4, PaO_2 14 kPa (108 mmHg). What is your management?

5 A young man with no past medical history comes to the Emergency Department having fallen off a ladder and hurt his left lower ribs. His observations are: alert, pulse 110/min, RR 24/min and BP 140/90 mmHg. You notice how clammy he is to touch. Could this man have a life-threatening haemorrhage?

6 A 50-year-old man weighing 70 kg with no past medical history is admitted with gastric outflow obstruction and is scheduled for surgery. His fluid balance chart for the past 24 h is as follows. Input: nil orally, 3 l i.v. 0.9% sodium chloride. Output: urine 500 ml total, bowels nil, nasogastric tube 4000 ml total. There are no i.v. antibiotics or other drugs and no fever is recorded. This morning's blood results show: Na 150 mmol/l, K 3.0 mmol/l, urea 12 mmol/l (33.3 mg/dl), creatinine 140 μmol/l (1.68 mg/dl). His BP and pulse are normal. What fluids should you prescribe for the next 24 h?

7 A patient comes back from theatre to your high-dependency area. His vital signs are: alert, pulse 80/min, BP 150/80 mmHg, RR 25/min, SpO_2 96% on 2 l oxygen via nasal cannulae and temperature 36°C. His arterial

blood gases show: pH 7.3, PaO$_2$ 15.0 (115 mmHg), PaCO$_2$ 4.0 (29 mmHg), st bicarbonate 15 mmol/l and BE −6. His CVP is 12 mmHg and he has cool hands and feet. He received Hartmann's and blood in theatre. How do you manage his acidosis?

8 A patient on ICU has been on maintenance crystalloid (0.9% saline) for several days and this morning's blood results show: Na 145 mmol/l, K 4.0 mmol/l, urea 4.5 mmol/l (12.5 mg/dl), creatinine 80 µmol/l (0.96 mg/dl). The patient is stable and the vital signs are normal. The arterial blood gases show: pH 7.3, PaO$_2$ 13.0 (100 mmHg), PaCO$_2$ 4.5 (34.6 mmHg), st bicarbonate 16 mmol/l and BE −5. The patient is doing well in every way and is expected to leave ICU in the next 24 h. The examination is normal. What is your management?

9 You have just put a CVP line into a patient who is unwell with a severe biliary infection. The CVP measures 15 mmHg. Should you give fluid?

10 You are asked to see an 80-year-old woman because she has a low BP. On examination her vital signs are: pulse 70/min, BP 90/60 mmHg, RR 14/min, SpO$_2$ 95% on air and temperature 37°C. She has warm hands and feet, feels well and is mobilising around the ward. What other parameters would you assess and what is your management?

Self-assessment: discussion

1 Management always starts with A (airway), B (breathing), C (circulation) and D (disability), as outlined in Chapter 1. This patient is both dehydrated (high sodium) and volume depleted (hypotension). He requires both water and volume expansion. Hypotonic 'maintenance fluid' should be prescribed, taking into account his water deficit, and colloid or 0.9% saline boluses can be given to expand his intravascular volume until either tissue perfusion is restored (see Box 5.2) or the patient starts to develop signs of fluid overload. As a rule, hypernatraemia should be corrected at the same rate in which it developed, in this case 2–3 days, because of the risk of cerebral pontine myelinolysis. In E (exposure and examination), a cause for his general deterioration should be sought. A likely cause is Gram-negative bacteraemia from his long-term catheter. The elderly commonly present with hypothermia and cool peripheries in sepsis.

2 Patients with decompensated liver disease typically have a low BP, and a low urea and creatinine. In this case, his urea and creatinine are higher than expected, although still within the 'normal' range. He also has a fever. Management in this case includes nasogastric feeding if his calorie intake is inadequate, expansion of intravascular volume with albumin or other colloid and Terlipressin for hepatorenal syndrome. Tense ascites can compromise the renal circulation and should be drained. Ascitic fluid should be analysed for spontaneous bacterial peritonitis, suggested by >250 neutrophils/mm^3. In this situation where there is hyponatraemia, sepsis and developing renal failure, hypotonic fluid should be avoided. Consult a liver specialist.

3 The history of recent major abdominal surgery makes fluid loss likely. This patient will probably have a positive balance on his fluid balance chart, but his third space losses cannot be measured. Look for other signs of volume depletion and cool extremities. He requires a fluid challenge and reassessment a short time later.

4 This patient is showing signs of hypoperfusion (i.e. cool peripheries, hypotension, oliguria and a metabolic acidosis). If the lungs are clear, a fluid challenge should still be given first, even in possible cardiogenic shock. This is because there is little point in trying to pharmacologically improve the contractility of a heart that is too empty to eject. The clinical response to a fluid challenge can be assessed immediately: Is there a rise in BP? This is an example of a situation where a CVP line would be used early, for close monitoring of fluid therapy and the administration of vaso-active drugs, dobutamine in this case. In cardiogenic shock causing severe hypotension (not due to surgical causes) dobutamine may not reverse hypoperfusion of vital organs because it increases CO, but does not necessarily raise BP. Aortic balloon pumping or vasopressors may be required.

5 Yes, healthy people have an intact sympathetic response to bleeding and are clammy and hypertensive as a result. Hypotension is a late sign. He has probably sustained a splenic injury.

6 The history, fluid balance chart and blood tests all point towards fluid loss and dehydration. Large gastric losses have resulted in hypokalaemia. He requires water and potassium. Water deficit can be calculated as follows:

Volume required (l) = $0.5 \times$ weight (kg) $\times$ ($Na^{2+} - 140$)/140.

This patient's water deficit is 2.5 l which can be given over the next 24 h as 5% dextrose, *in addition* to his ongoing maintenance requirements and anticipated losses, which can be given as Hartmann's solution. At least 4 l of Hartmann's is required over the next 24 h, and this should contain enough replacement potassium as well, though this should be guided by repeat blood tests.

7 This patient has signs of hypoperfusion (i.e. cool peripheries), increased RR and metabolic acidosis. The history points towards fluid loss. A CVP of 12 mmHg in this context does not mean that the patient has had enough fluid. Give a fluid challenge and assess the response both clinically and in terms of the CVP.

8 If the patient has no clinical signs of hypoperfusion and the anion gap or lactate is normal, this mild metabolic acidosis is most likely a hyperchloraemic acidosis caused by prolonged infusion of 0.9% saline. You could switch the patient to a more balanced solution (e.g. Hartmann's).

9 The history of sepsis points towards volume depletion. What is the clinical assessment of the patient? Use this and not a single CVP reading to guide your next course of action. Give a fluid challenge and assess the response.

10 Hypotension does not necessarily mean hypoperfusion. You could assess for signs of this (see Box 5.2) and also look at her medication chart. Some people normally have a low BP which does not cause problems with organ perfusion. There is no 'normal' BP. What matters is perfusion.

References

1. Gosling P. Salt of the earth or a drop in the ocean? A pathophysiological approach to fluid resuscitation. *Emergency Medical Journal* 2003; **20**: 306–315. This article can be downloaded free at www.emj.bmjjournals.com
2. Guha IN and Sheron N. Managing fluid balance in patients with liver disease. *Acute Medicine* 2004; **3(3)**: 110–113.
3. Sort P, Navasa M, Arroyo V *et al.* Effect of intravenous albumin on renal impairment and mortality in patients with cirrhosis and spontaneous bacterial peritonitis. *New England Journal of Medicine* 1999; **341**: 403–409.
4. Moreau R, Durand F, Pynard T *et al.* Terlipressin in patients with cirrhosis and type 1 hepatorenal syndrome: a retrospective multicentre study. *Gastroenterology* 2002; **122**: 923–930.
5. Kaplan LJ, McPartland K, Santora TA and Trooskin SZ. Start with a subjective assessment of skin temperature to identify hypoperfusion in ICU patients. *Journal of Trauma-Injury Infection and Critical Care* 2001; **50**: 620–627.
6. ATLS courses (Advanced Trauma and Life Support) are run by the Royal College of Surgeons of England and Edinburgh and focus on trauma care. www.rcseng.ac.uk/courses (under basic surgical training).
7. Dellinger RP, Carlet J, Masur H *et al.* Surviving sepsis campaign guidelines for the management of severe sepsis and septic shock. *Critical Care Medicine* 2004; **32(3)**: 858–872.
8. Harvey S, Harrison D, Singer M *et al.* Assessment of the clinical effectiveness of pulmonary artery catheters in management of patients in intensive care (PAC-Man): a randomised controlled trial. *Lancet* 2005; **366**: 472–477.
9. Williams EL, Hildebrand KL, McCormick SA and Bedel MJ. The effect of intravenous Lactated Ringer's solution vs 0.9% sodium chloride solution on serum osmolality in human volunteers. *Anesthesia and Analgesia* 1999; **88**: 999–1003.
10. Cochrane Injuries Group Albumin Reviewers. Human albumin administration in critically ill patients: systematic review of randomised controlled trials. *British Medical Journal* 1998; **317**: 235–240.
11. The SAFE Study Investigators. A comparison of albumin and saline for fluid resuscitation in the intensive care unit. *New England Journal of Medicine* 2004; **350**: 2247–2256.
12. Hebert PC, Wells G, Blajchman MA, Marshall J, Martin C, Pagliarello G, Tweeddale M, Schweitzer I and Yetisir E. A multicenter, randomized, controlled clinical trial of transfusion requirements in critical care. Transfusion Requirements in Critical Care Investigators, Canadian Critical Care Trials Group. *New England Journal of Medicine* 1999, **340**, 409–417.
13. Corwin HL, Gettinger A, Pearl RG *et al.* The CRIT study: anaemia and blood transfusion in the critically ill – current clinical practice in the United States. *Critical Care Medicine* 2004; **32**: 39–52.

14. Vincent JL, Baron JF, Reinhart K *et al*. ABC (anaemia and blood transfusion in critical care) investigators. Anaemia and blood transfusion in critically ill patients. *Journal of the American Medical Association* 2002; **288**: 1499–1507.
15. Roberts I, Alderson P, Bunn F, Ker K and Schierhout G. Colloids versus crystalloids for fluid resuscitation in critically ill patients. *The Cochrane Database of Systemic Reviews* 2004; **18(4)**: CD000567.

Further resource

• Park GR and Roe PG. *Fluid Balance and Volume Resuscitation for Beginners*. Greenwich Medical Media, London, 2000.

CHAPTER 6

Sepsis

By the end of this chapter you will be able to:

- Know the definitions of sepsis
- Understand the basic pathophysiology of sepsis
- Be aware of the Surviving Sepsis Campaign and its recommendations
- Understand the principles of early goal directed therapy
- Know how inotropes and vasopressors work
- Appreciate the effects of sepsis on the lung
- Apply this to your clinical practice

The incidence of sepsis is increasing [1] and it is a major cause of morbidity and mortality in hospital. Around one third of UK ICU admissions are now due to severe sepsis where it is the leading cause of death. In the USA, sepsis causes more deaths than acute myocardial infarction or lung cancer and costs $17 billion each year in hospital costs [2]. With standard supportive care alone, mortality remains unacceptably high, increasing with the number of failing organs [3] (see Fig. 6.1). However, early identification and appropriate treatment of sepsis improves patient outcome.

Definitions

In 1991, the American College of Chest Physicians and the Society of Critical Care Medicine convened a consensus conference in order to provide a practical

Number of failing organs	Percentage of ICU patients	Percentage mortality
0	35.1	3.2
1	24.9	10.6
2	16.8	25.5
3	12.1	51.4
4	6.5	61.3
5	3.0	67.4
6	1.6	91.3

Figure 6.1 Mortality of sepsis on ICU according to the number of failing organs.

framework and define the spectrum of sepsis [4]. In 2003, the International Sepsis Definitions Conference expanded on these definitions [5]. A simplified version is shown in Fig. 6.2. You will notice that the term 'septicaemia' is not used.

Other important terms include 'systemic inflammatory response syndrome' (SIRS) and 'multiple organ dysfunction syndrome' (MODS). SIRS is clinically identical to sepsis and severe sepsis, except that it is caused by a variety of insults including trauma, major surgery, pancreatitis and burns as well as infection. This overlap is illustrated in Fig. 6.3. The term MODS is a clinical syndrome in which progressive and potentially reversible dysfunction in two or more organ systems occur. It is also induced by a variety of acute insults but its occurrence in sepsis is characteristic.

	Definition
Infection	Invasion of micro-organisms into a normally sterile site, often associated with an inflammatory host response
Bacteraemia	Viable bacteria in the bloodstream
Sepsis	Clinical evidence of infection plus a systemic response indicated by two or more of the following: • Hyper- (>38°C) or hypothermia (<36°C) • Tachycardia (heart rate >90/min) • Tachypnoea (respiratory rate >20/min) • White blood cells >12 × 10^9 or <4 × 10^9 or 'left shift'
Severe sepsis	Sepsis associated with organ dysfunction*: • Hypotension • Poor urine output • Hypoxaemia • Confusion • Metabolic (lactic) acidosis • Disseminated intravascular coagulation
Septic shock	Severe sepsis with hypotension unresponsive to intravascular volume replacement with fluids
Refractory shock	Hypotension not responding to vaso-active drugs

Figure 6.2 Definitions in the sepsis continuum. *Other organ dysfunctions include: ileus, abnormal liver tests and mottled skin.

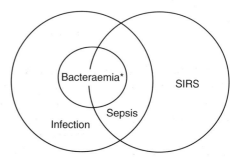

Figure 6.3 SIRS and sepsis.
*Fungaemia and parasitaemia also occur.

Basic pathophysiology of sepsis

The features seen in severe sepsis are a result of the body's over-response to infection. There is an uncontrolled cascade of inflammation, coagulation and impaired fibrinolysis. The microcirculation is disrupted, leading to tissue hypoxia and organ dysfunction. Severe sepsis is a complicated disease and the subject of much research.

Inflammation

The body's initial response to a pro-inflammatory insult is to release mediators like tumour necrosis factor, interleukin 1, interleukin 6 and platelet-activating factor. These mediators have multiple overlapping effects designed to repair existing damage and limit new damage. To ensure that the effects of the pro-inflammatory mediators do not become destructive, the body then launches compensatory anti-inflammatory mediators like interleukin 4 and interleukin 10 which down-regulate the initial pro-inflammatory response. In severe sepsis, regulation of the early response to a pro-inflammatory insult is lost and a massive systemic reaction occurs with excessive or inappropriate inflammatory reactions resulting in the development of diffuse capillary injury.

Coagulation/impaired fibrinolysis

Inflammatory mediators promote coagulation. Clots form in the microcirculation (capillaries) leading to impaired blood flow which can be demonstrated by research imaging techniques [6]. This leads to tissue hypoxia and organ dysfunction. Coagulation and fibrinolysis are usually finely balanced but the fibrinolytic system is suppressed in sepsis.

Inappropriate activation of the coagulation cascade results in widespread fibrin deposition (clot formation) and coagulation factors and platelets are consumed faster than they can be replaced. Hence the paradox of both microvascular thrombosis and bleeding, a condition known as disseminated intravascular coagulation (DIC).

Therefore, the following laboratory changes are seen in severe sepsis:
- Reduced platelets
- Prolonged activated partial thromboplastin time (APTT), prothrombin time (PT) and thrombin time (TT)
- Reduced fibrinogen
- Elevated D-dimer
- Microangiopathic haemolysis leading to anaemia and reticulocytosis.

Disruption of the microcirculation

The normal role of the endothelium includes interaction with leucocytes, the release of cytokines and inflammatory mediators, the release of mediators which vasodilate or vasoconstrict and taking part in the coagulation system. In severe sepsis there is physical as well as chemical dysfunction of the endothelium. Holes literally appear which lead to capillary leak causing hypovolaemia and oedema.

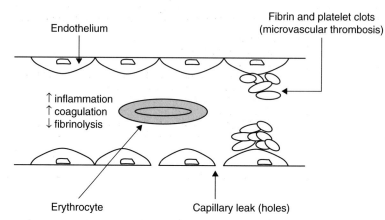

Figure 6.4 The pathophysiology of severe sepsis. Microvascular thrombosis and endothelial dysfunction lead to tissue hypoxia.

To summarise, microvascular hypoperfusion occurs in severe sepsis as a result of inflammation, coagulation abnormalities and disruption of the microcirculation. This is diagrammatically represented in Fig. 6.4.

Clinical features

The clinical features of severe sepsis are the result of the pathophysiological features described above:
- A systemic inflammatory response (Fig. 6.2)
- Reduced systemic vascular resistance (SVR) or vasodilatation
- Increased capillary permeability
- Coagulopathy with microvascular thrombosis
- Metabolic (lactic) acidosis
- Organ dysfunction (Fig. 6.2).

Although the 'typical' patient with severe sepsis has a fever, tachycardia, high respiratory rate and vasodilatation, *many patients do not have these features.* The elderly or immunosuppressed may simply present with hypotension and can be 'shut down'. Severe sepsis can also cause myocardial dysfunction due to circulating toxins, acidosis and hypoxaemia. Sepsis is a dynamic process with evolution of physical signs and a continuum of physiological responses.

Treatment of severe sepsis aims to maximise oxygen delivery to the tissues, control the underlying infection and interrupt the pathophysiological processes described above.

Surviving sepsis

The Surviving Sepsis Campaign (SSC) was formed in 2002 as a collaboration of the European Society of Intensive Care Medicine, International Sepsis Forum and the Society of Critical Care Medicine [7]. It was established to improve the

1. Resuscitation	Begin immediately and accomplish within 6 h of presentation:
	
	• Lactate measured
	• Blood cultures performed
	• Broad-spectrum antibiotics within 1 h
	• Treat hypotension or elevated lactate with fluid challenges
	• If hypotension or elevated lactate present:
	   (i) Aim for central venous pressure (CVP) >8 mmHg
	   (ii) And urine output >0.5 ml/kg/h
	   (iii) Treat ongoing hypotension with vasopressors
	   (iv) Aim for central venous SaO$_2$ of >70%
	
	Ongoing care in ICU

2. Management*	Consider immediately and accomplish within 24 h of presentation: • Control blood glucose • Administer low-dose steroids in patients requiring vasopressors • Consider activated protein C (APC) therapy • Ventilate with low inspiratory plateau pressures

Figure 6.5 Guidelines for the management of severe sepsis in adults. *Additional management includes locating the source of infection and DVT prophylaxis. The SSC guidance also discusses sedation and neuromuscular blockade, stress ulcer prophylaxis, when to administer blood products and the choice of vasopressors/inotropes.

diagnosis, management and treatment of sepsis. One of the main goals of this initiative is to reduce the mortality of sepsis by 25% within 5 years through education and the implementation of evidence-based guidelines [8]. Deaths from acute myocardial infarction have been reduced from 25%–30% to 8% over the past 20 years as a result of new pharmacological and mechanical interventions together with improvements in supportive care. The management of patients with sepsis is now beginning to receive the same level of intense clinical commitment as was shown to acute myocardial infarction in the late 1980s.

Of particular importance is the fact that the outcome from sepsis can be improved by simple interventions outside the ICU. Early recognition and treatment of sepsis is vital if organ dysfunction and death is to be prevented. The US Institute for Healthcare Improvement has distilled the SSC guidelines into 'bundles' for hospitals to implement and audit [9]. A bundle is a group of interventions that, when executed together, result in better outcomes than when implemented individually. The individual bundle elements are evidence based. There are two sepsis bundles, the resuscitation bundle and the management bundle. A summary is shown in Fig. 6.5.

Resuscitation

A high lactate (>4 mmol/l) is often present in severe sepsis, due to tissue hypoxia and anaerobic metabolism. A persistently raised lactate is a poor prognostic indicator [10]. Although a high lactate can be due to other reasons (e.g. reduced clearance by the liver), any patient with sepsis and an elevated lactate should enter the sepsis resuscitation bundle (Fig. 6.5) even if the BP is not low. Many arterial blood gas analysers measure serum lactate. Sometimes lactate may not be raised despite a metabolic acidosis with no other explanation apart from sepsis. In this situation, enter the sepsis resuscitation bundle in the same way.

Blood samples should be obtained as the patient is being cannulated for the administration of i.v. fluid. At least two sets of blood cultures should be taken with at least 10 ml in each bottle, as this increases the yield [11]. *Do not wait for a pyrexia before taking blood culture samples.* Pyrexia is only one indicator of severe sepsis and some patients may be hypothermic. Samples should also be sent for culture as soon as possible from any other potential source of infection: intravascular devices, urine, wounds, sputum and cerebrospinal fluid.

Broad-spectrum i.v. antibiotics should be administered (not just prescribed) within the first hour after recognition of severe sepsis. Antibiotic therapy will be tailored at 48–72 h depending on the results of cultures. The choice of broad spectrum antibiotic depends on the likely source of sepsis and local guidelines. Early antibiotic administration reduces mortality in patients with bacterial infections [12]. The main sources of infection in severe sepsis are the chest and abdomen (including the urinary tract). A table of the commonly used first line antibiotics in the UK is shown in Fig. 6.6.

Hypotension or an elevated lactate should be aggressively treated. The goals of resuscitation are to restore intravascular volume, improve organ perfusion (with vasopressors and/or inotropes if necessary) and maximise oxygen delivery. The principle of oxygen delivery was described in Chapter 2 in simple terms, but will be expanded further below.

In most tissues, oxygen consumption (VO_2) is determined by metabolic demand and does not rely on oxygen delivery (DO_2). But if oxygen delivery is reduced to a critical level, oxygen consumption becomes 'supply dependent'. In severe sepsis, the tissues become supply dependent at higher levels of oxygen delivery. This is shown diagrammatically in Fig. 6.7. Oxygen demand increases in sepsis but oxygen delivery is impaired by the pathophysiological changes taking place in both the macro- and the micro-circulation. In the macrocirculation these are hypovolaemia, vaso-regulatory dysfunction and myocardial depression. The abnormalities in the microcirculation have already been described. These changes combine to induce global tissue hypoxia, anaerobic metabolism and lactic acidosis. In addition, it is likely that abnormal cell function also contributes to tissue hypoxia in severe sepsis [13].

Early goal directed therapy

Early goal directed therapy (EGDT) is based on the early recognition of this DO_2/VO_2 imbalance and was described in an article by Rivers *et al* [14]. The SSC guidelines state that the resuscitation of a patient with severe sepsis should begin as soon as the syndrome is recognised and should not be delayed until

Symptoms and signs	Likely organisms	Intravenous therapy
Severe community-acquired pneumonia	*Pneumococcus, Mycoplasma, Legionella*	Cefuroxime + erythromycin (high-dose erythromycin ± rifampicin for *Legionella*)
Hospital-acquired pneumonia	*S. aureus*, mixed anaerobes, Gram-negative rods	Cefuroxime (take into account antibiotic/ICU history and sputum cultures)
Intra-abdominal sepsis (e.g. post-operative or peritonitis)	Gram-negative bacteria, anaerobes	Cefuroxime and metronidazole ± gentamicin
Pyelonephritis	*E. coli*, Enterobacter	Cefuroxime or ciprofloxacin
Meningitis	*Pneumococcus, Meningococcus*	High-dose cefotaxime
Meningitis aged over 55	*Pneumococcus, Meningococcus, Listeria*, Gram-negative rods	High-dose cefotaxime + ampicillin
Neutropenic patient (e.g. chemotherapy)	*S. aureus, Pseudomonas, Klebsiella, E. coli*	Piperacillin–tazobactam + gentamicin
Line infections	*S. aureus*, Gram-negative bacteria	Replace line if possible; vancomycin or flucloxacillin + gentamicin
Bone – osteomyelitis or septic arthritis	*S. aureus*	Flucloxacillin ± fucidic acid
Acute endocarditis	*S. aureus*, Gram-negative bacteria, *S. viridans*	Benzylpenicillin + gentamicin
Returning traveller	Seek advice from an expert because of resistant strains	

Figure 6.6 First line antibiotics in the UK. Note: If serious penicillin or cephalosporin allergy, consult urgently with an expert (e.g. consultant in microbiology).

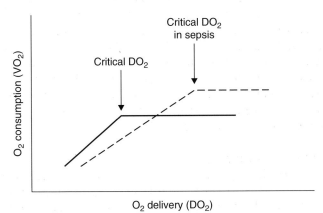

Figure 6.7 The relationship between oxygen consumption and oxygen delivery in sepsis.

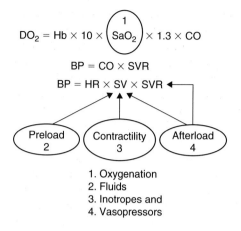

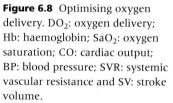

1. Oxygenation
2. Fluids
3. Inotropes and
4. Vasopressors

Figure 6.8 Optimising oxygen delivery. DO_2: oxygen delivery; Hb: haemoglobin; SaO_2: oxygen saturation; CO: cardiac output; BP: blood pressure; SVR: systemic vascular resistance and SV: stroke volume.

admission to the ICU. Although severe sepsis is an ICU disease, it has been shown that optimising oxygen delivery with EGDT during the pre-intensive care period reduces morbidity and mortality rates significantly.

The oxygen delivery equation is shown in Fig. 6.8, with the subcomponents of cardiac output (CO) illustrated. Now the basis of resuscitation can be understood, indeed the basis of intensive care medicine, in terms of oxygen delivery: oxygenation, fluids and inotropes/vasopressors.

Rivers *et al.* aimed to normalise oxygen delivery by optimising preload (using central venous pressure (CVP) monitoring), afterload (using mean arterial pressure, MAP) and contractility (guided by central venous oxygen saturation ($ScvO_2$), which has been shown to be a surrogate for CO [15]). They randomised patients arriving at an urban emergency department with severe sepsis to receive either usual care or EGDT. There were 130 patients in each group and there were no significant differences in baseline characteristics. All patients received continuous monitoring of vital signs, blood tests, antibiotics, urinary catheterisation, arterial and central venous catheterisation. The control group received usual care which was to maintain CVP 8–12 mmHg, MAP above 65 mmHg and urine output of at least 0.5 ml/kg/h. These goals were achieved with fluid boluses and vasopressors if required.

The EGDT group had slightly different goals: CVP 8–12 mmHg, MAP 65–90 mmHg, urine output of at least 0.5 ml/kg/h and central venous oxygen saturation ($ScvO_2$) of at least 70%. These goals were achieved with fluid boluses, vasopressors or vasodilators, and if the $ScvO_2$ was low, red cells were transfused to achieve a haematocrit of at least 30% and dobutamine was given if necessary. If these goals were not achieved, patients were sedated and mechanically ventilated to reduce oxygen demand.

All patients were transferred to an ICU after 6 h where the physicians were blinded to the patient's assigned group. Patients were followed for 60 days. The study found that hospital mortality was reduced in the EGDT group

(30.5% vs 46.5%). Hospital stay was also shorter and there was less incidence of sudden cardiovascular collapse (10.3% vs 21%) and progression to multiple organ failure (16.2% vs 21.8%). During the period of initial resuscitation, patients in the EGDT group received significantly more fluids, red cell transfusions and inotropes. A *post-hoc* analysis showed that patients who had evidence of persisting global tissue hypoxia despite a normal BP (indicated by a reduced ScvO$_2$ and elevated lactate) had a higher mortality than those who received EGDT. After 6 h of therapy, 39.8% of the control group vs 5.1% of the EGDT group had persisting global tissue hypoxia.

The above explains why the sepsis resuscitation guidelines include the maintenance of adequate ScvO$_2$ as a goal. Rivers *et al.* achieved this by using oxygen therapy, red cell transfusion if necessary, dobutamine and mechanical ventilation. However, only 18 out of the 130 patients in the EGDT group received dobutamine in the first 6 h and the outcome of this subset is not stated. It is unclear at the present time whether or not this element of the SSC guidelines is truly evidence based.

Mixed SvO$_2$ is obtained from mixed venous blood in the right ventricle via a pulmonary artery (PA) catheter. It is used as an indicator of oxygen supply and demand in critically ill patients. The normal value is around 75% and tissue oxygen delivery is considered critical below 50%. It is a surrogate marker, because it is related to arterial oxygen content, oxygen consumption and CO. ScvO$_2$ can be measured using a central line, either by a catheter capable of doing so, or by drawing central venous blood and measuring oxygen saturation (SaO$_2$) on a blood gas machine. The normal value is around 70%.

Septic shock as defined by hypotension is a simplistic and perhaps outdated concept. The early recognition of global tissue hypoxia despite a normal BP can occur in the emergency department or on a general ward. The patient may have signs of sepsis or a systemic inflammatory response (see Fig. 6.2) with a lactic acidosis. Such patients require resuscitation.

The haemodynamic goals of resuscitation in sepsis are to maintain the MAP above 65 mmHg and the CVP above 8 mmHg using fluids and vasopressors. Sepsis needs to be treated with *successive fluid boluses*. An initial bolus of 20 ml/kg of crystalloid is suggested, or the colloid equivalent. Fluid resuscitation, which fluid to use and the interpretation of CVP has been discussed in Chapter 5. MAP is the average arterial BP throughout the cardiac cycle and is a more useful term when considering tissue perfusion. It can be calculated as approximately (2 $\times$ diastolic) + systolic divided by 3.

Further management

Following the initial resuscitation phase, further management includes control of blood glucose. Hyperglycaemia is a common finding in critical illness, caused by insulin resistance in the liver and muscles in order to provide glucose for the brain and other vital functions. Intensive insulin therapy to maintain blood glucose within the normal range has been shown to significantly reduce mortality in critically ill patients. In one study, the incidence of bacteraemia, acute renal failure, critical illness polyneuropathy and blood transfusion was also halved [16].

In patients with severe sepsis, there are complex effects on the hypothalamic–pituitary–adrenal axis, including relative adrenal insufficiency. Corticosteroids are known to have effects on vascular tone as well as anti-inflammatory actions. The use of low-dose corticosteroids (50 mg of i.v. hydrocortisone four times a day) has been shown to reduce mortality and dependence on vasopressors. A Cochrane meta-analysis of randomised controlled trials of low-dose corticosteroids in patients with septic shock showed that 28-day all-cause mortality was reduced [17]. The number needed to treat with low-dose corticosteroids to save one additional life was nine. Treatment with low-dose corticosteroids was also more likely to reverse shock (dependence on vasopressors). High-dose corticosteroids have not been shown to be beneficial and may even be harmful.

A short synacthen test is useful in identifying 'responders' from 'non-responders', but should not delay the administration of corticosteroids. Dexamethasone (8 mg i.v.) can be administered pending a short synacthen test if needed, as this does not interfere with the test. A responder is defined as a patient with an increase in cortisol of 250 nmol/l (9 μg/dl) or more 30–60 min after the administration of i.v. synacthen (ACTH). Some experts would discontinue corticosteroid therapy in responders as treatment may be ineffective in this group.

Drotrecogin Alfa (Activated), or recombinant activated protein C (APC), inhibits the generation of thrombin via inactivation of factor Va and VIIIa. It also has profibrinolytic and anti-inflammatory activity. Significant decreases in APC have been documented in severe sepsis. A large-multicentre randomised controlled trial (PROWESS) [18] showed that recombinant APC reduced mortality in patients with severe sepsis (24.7% vs 30.8%). However, the incidence of serious bleeding was higher in the APC group (3.5% vs 2%), especially in patients with risk factors for bleeding.

A further international clinical trial of APC in 2378 patients with severe sepsis (ENHANCE) [19] showed that the mortality rate was lower for patients treated within 24 h of organ dysfunction compared with those treated after the first 24 h (33% vs 41%). The results also indicated that early treatment with APC reduced length of stay on the ICU. A subgroup of 872 patients with multiple organ dysfunction enrolled in another international multicentre randomised controlled trial (ADDRESS) [20] showed that mortality was unchanged in patients with sepsis and single organ failure treated with APC.

At the present time, APC is recommended for early treatment of severe sepsis in adults with more than one organ failure. Each ICU works to local guidelines. APC is administered by continuous i.v. infusion for a total of 96 h on an ICU. The National Institute of Clinical Excellence (NICE) UK recommends that it may only be administered by a specialist in intensive care medicine. The contraindications to APC use are shown in Box 6.1.

Box 6.1 Contraindications to the use of recombinant APC

Decisions must be made on an individual basis as a contraindication to APC therapy may be relative to the risk of death from severe sepsis. Patients who have most to gain have two or more failing organ systems and an APACHE 2 (Acute Physiological And Chronic Health Evaluation) score >25.

Example contraindications
- Currently anticoagulated or recent thrombolysis
- Active bleeding or coagulopathy
- Platelet count <30
- Recent major surgery
- Recent gastrointestinal bleed (6 weeks)
- Chronic liver disease
- Recent haemorrhagic stroke (3 months)
- Recent cranial or spinal procedure or head injury (2 months)
- Trauma with risk of bleeding
- Epidural catheter *in situ*
- Intracranial tumour
- Known hypersensitivity to APC
- Moribund and likely to die
- Pancreatitis and chronic renal failure were also excluded from the PROWESS study.

Inotropes and vasopressors

An inotrope is an agent that increases myocardial contractility. A vasopressor is an agent that vasoconstricts and increases SVR. A vaso-active drug is a generic term meaning either. To recap from Chapter 5, BP = CO × SVR. CO = heart rate × stroke volume and stroke volume depends on preload, contractility and afterload. This basic physiology is clinically important because the treatment of hypoperfusion has to follow a logical sequence. There is little point in trying to pharmacologically improve the contractility of a heart that is too empty to eject.

BP measurements with a cuff are unreliable at low BPs. Ideally, BP is measured using an arterial line, which also measures MAP. An MAP of <60 mmHg is associated with compromised autoregulation in the coronary, renal and cerebral circulations. As a practical guide for the wards, aim for a systolic BP >90 mmHg, or one that adequately perfuses the vital organs. This may be higher in patients who usually have hypertension.

Invasive or more sophisticated monitoring than simply pulse, BP, and urine output should be instituted early in severe sepsis. Unlike other causes of shock, the CO is often maintained or even increased in severe sepsis. Hypotension results from alterations in the distribution of blood flow and a low SVR. SVR can be measured by a PA catheter, oesophageal doppler and other systems described in Chapter 5, and is of great value in titrating vasopressors in severe sepsis. SVR may be thought of as the resistance against which the heart pumps and is mainly determined by the diameter of arterioles. It is calculated as follows:

$$SVR = MAP - CVP \text{ (mmHg)} \times 80 \text{ (correction factor)}/CO \text{ (l/min)}.$$

The normal range is 1000–1500 dyn s/cm^5.

Receptors in the circulation

In order to understand how inotropes and vasopressors work, it is important to know about the main types of receptor in the circulation. These adrenoreceptors act via G proteins and cyclic AMP at the cellular level. Fig. 6.9 shows the action of various receptors in the circulation and the action of commonly used vaso-active drugs.

All the drugs below are short acting and their effects on the circulation are seen immediately.

Norepinephrine (noradrenaline)

Norepinephrine is a potent α-agonist (vasoconstrictor), raising BP by increasing SVR. It has a little β1-receptor activity causing increased contractility, heart rate and CO but it has no effect on β2-receptors. It acts mainly as a vasopressor, with little inotropic effect. Through vasoconstriction, norepinephrine reduces

Receptor	Action	Where
α-receptors	Vasoconstriction	Peripheral, renal, coronary
β1-receptors	↑ Contractility ↑ Heart rate ↑ Cardiac output	Heart
β2-receptors	Vasodilatation	Peripheral, renal
DA (dopamine) receptors	Range of actions (see later)	Renal, gut, coronary

Vaso-active drug	α	β1	β2	DA
Norepinephrine (noradrenaline)	+++	+		
Dopamine – Low dose – Medium dose – High dose	 ++	 ++ ++	 + +	 +++ ++ +
Dobutamine		+++	++	
Epinephrine (adrenaline)	+ to +++	+++	++	
Dopexamine		+	+++	++

Figure 6.9 Receptors in the circulation and the action of common vaso-active drugs.

renal, gut and muscle perfusion but in patients with severe sepsis, it increases renal and gut perfusion by increasing perfusion pressure.

Dopamine
Dopamine stimulates adrenoreceptors and dopaminergic receptors. The effects of dopamine change with increasing dose:
- At low doses the predominant effects are those of dopaminergic stimulation causing an increase in renal and gut blood flow.
- At medium doses, β1-receptor effects predominate causing increased myocardial contractility, heart rate and CO.
- At high doses, α-stimulation predominates causing an increase in SVR and reduction in renal blood flow. High doses of dopamine are associated with arrhythmias and increased myocardial oxygen demand.

There is marked individual variation in plasma levels of dopamine in the critically ill, making it difficult to know which effects are predominating. Dopamine may accumulate in patients with hepatic dysfunction.

Dobutamine
Dobutamine has predominant β1-effects which increases heart rate and contractility and hence CO. It also has β2-effects which reduce systemic and pulmonary vascular resistance. Mild α-effects may be unmasked in a patient on β-blockers (because of down regulation). The increase in myocardial oxygen consumption from dobutamine administration is offset by the reduction in afterload that also occurs. These properties make dobutamine a logical first choice inotrope in ischaemic cardiac failure. Dobutamine has no effect on visceral vascular beds but increased renal and splanchnic flow occur as a result of increased CO. The increase in CO may increase BP but since SVR is reduced or unchanged, the effect of dobutamine on BP is variable. Dobutamine is the pharmacological agent of choice to increase CO when this is depressed in septic shock.

Epinephrine (adrenaline)
Epinephrine is a potent β1-, β2- and α-agonist. The cardiovascular effects of epinephrine depend on dose. At lower doses, β1-stimulation predominates (i.e. increased contractility, heart rate and hence CO). There is some stimulation of β2-receptors (which also cause bronchodilatation) but this does not predominate and therefore BP increases. α-stimulation becomes more predominant with increasing doses leading to vasoconstriction which further increases systolic BP. Renal and gut vasoconstriction also occurs. There is a greater increase in myocardial oxygen consumption than seen with dobutamine. Metabolic effects include a fall in plasma potassium, a rise in serum glucose and stimulation of metabolism which can lead to a rise in serum lactate.

Dopexamine
Dopexamine is a synthetic analogue of dopamine without α effects. It is a β2-agonist with one third of the potency of dopamine on DA1 receptors.

Dopexamine causes an increase in heart rate and CO as well as causing peripheral vasodilatation and an increase in renal and splanchnic blood flow. CO is increased as a result of afterload reduction and mild inotropy. In comparison to other inotropes, dopexamine causes less increase in myocardial oxygen consumption. Dopexamine may have some anti-inflammatory activity, but its main focus of interest has been on its ability to improve renal, gut and hepatic blood flow which is thought to be beneficial in preserving gastrointestinal mucosal integrity in certain patients.

Mini-tutorial: dopamine or noradrenaline in sepsis?

According to the SSC guidelines, a vasopressor should be commenced if the patient remains hypotensive after two fluid boluses (or a total of 40ml/kg crystalloid) regardless of CVP measurements. The rationale behind this is that vital organ perfusion is threatened by severe hypotension, even while fluid therapy is taking place. In inexperienced hands, the administration of vasopressors before fluids could be detrimental. Vasopressors can worsen organ perfusion in a volume-depleted patient, raising BP at the expense of vital organ perfusion (e.g. the kidneys and gut). An unnecessarily high BP can be particularly harmful. Therefore, a vasopressor should only be started by an expert while proper fluid resuscitation is taking place.

Dopamine or norepinephrine (noradrenaline) are first choice vasopressors in severe sepsis. In the past, there were concerns that norepinephrine may vasoconstrict the gut and renal circulation leading to detrimental effects. But in patients with sepsis, this appears not to be the case [21,22]. One particular study showed that norepinephrine use is associated with better outcome compared to dopamine in patients with severe sepsis [23].

Norepinephrine appears to be more effective at reversing hypotension in severe sepsis [24]. One prospective, double-blind, randomised trial compared norepinephrine and dopamine in the treatment of septic shock, defined by hypotension despite adequate fluid replacement, with a low SVR, high CO, oliguria and lactic acidosis. Patients with similar characteristics were assigned to receive either norepinephrine or dopamine. If the haemodynamic and metabolic abnormalities were not corrected with the maximum dose of one drug then the other was added. Only 31% patients were successfully treated with dopamine compared with 93% with norepinephrine; 10 of the 11 patients who did not respond to dopamine and remained hypotensive and oliguric were successfully treated with norepinephrine. The authors conclude that norepinephrine was more effective and reliable than dopamine in reversing the abnormalities of septic shock.

Current practice in the UK, therefore, is to use norepinephrine (noradrenaline) as the first line vasopressor for severe sepsis and to add dobutamine if a low CO is also present. Epinephrine (adrenaline) is not generally recommended in the treatment of severe sepsis because of its effects on the gut and it is more likely to cause tachycardias. In addition, its metabolic effects can increase lactate and so this surrogate marker of perfusion may be lost.

Other vaso-active drugs used in sepsis

Vasopressin is an option if hypotension is refractory to other vasopressors. It is a direct vasoconstrictor that acts on vasopressin receptors in the vasculature. In vasodilatory shock, vasopressin levels are inappropriately low due to reduced production by the pituitary gland.

Methylene blue can be useful in elevating BP in refractory shock. It acts by inhibiting guanylate cyclase. Nitric oxide stimulates guanylate cyclase to produce vasodilatation and reduced responsiveness to catecholamines. Methylene blue thus increases vascular tone.

The effects of sepsis on the lung

The inflammation and microcirculatory changes that take place in sepsis also affect the lung. Respiratory dysfunction ranges from subclinical disease to acute lung injury (ALI) to acute respiratory distress syndrome (ARDS). ARDS can be caused by a variety of insults, but is common in sepsis; 50% of patients with severe sepsis develop ALI or ARDS. Patients with ALI/ARDS have bilateral patchy infiltrates on the chest X-ray and a low PaO_2 to FiO_2 ratio, which is not due to fluid overload or heart failure [25].

The pathological changes in ARDS are divided into three phases:

1 The early exudative phase (days 1–5) characterised by oedema and haemorrhage.
2 The fibro-proliferative phase (days 6–10) characterised by organisation and repair.
3 The fibrotic phase (after 10 days) characterised by fibrosis.

The hallmark of ARDS is alveolar epithelial inflammation, air space flooding with plasma proteins, surfactant depletion and loss of normal endothelial reactivity. In ALI/ARDS, compensatory hypoxic vasoconstriction is impaired, leading to shunting of blood through non-ventilated areas of lung. Refractory hypoxaemia therefore occurs. There is also increased airway resistance and reduced thoracic compliance. The development of ARDS complicates the management of severe sepsis. Oxygenation is important, but high ventilation pressures can cause more lung damage and also have detrimental effects on the systemic circulation.

Research into ARDS has led to several different lung protection strategies, including better fluid management, different ways of ventilating patients and the use of steroids in non-resolving ARDS. Ventilating patients with ALI/ARDS using smaller tidal volumes and lower peak inspiratory pressures in sepsis improves outcome [26]. The modest hypercapnia which results is thought to be safe. Therefore the SSC guidelines recommend ventilating patients with severe sepsis using lower tidal volumes (6 ml/kg) with inspiratory plateau pressures <30 cmH_2O. The rationale for this is that mechanical ventilation, through shear forces and barotrauma, can perpetuate the inflammation and lung damage which is part of the process in ARDS.

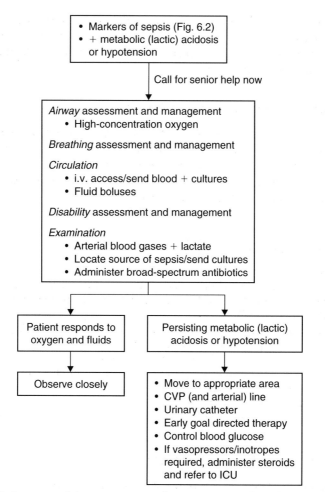

Figure 6.10 Summary of the management of severe sepsis (within 6 h of presentation).

Other treatments in sepsis

Plasmapheresis has been studied and is sometimes used in severe sepsis as a means of removing toxic mediators from the circulation and replacing immunoglobulins and clotting factors. At the present time, there is not enough evidence for this to be recommended as a routine treatment.

Compromised gut perfusion leads to breakdown of the mucosal barrier and bacteria translocate into the circulation where they stimulate cytokine production, inflammation and organ dysfunction. This theory has been demonstrated in animal studies, but the role of 'bacterial gut translocation' in the development of multiple organ failure in humans is still an area of research. All the inotropes used in sepsis have been studied with regard to their effect on the splanchnic circulation for this reason. Nutritional support (via naso-gastric tube) is considered important in severe sepsis to help maintain gut mucosal integrity, as well as to prevent stress ulcers and provide nutrition in this hypercatabolic state.

Approach to the patient with sepsis

Armed with the knowledge of the pathophysiology of sepsis, the rationale for EGDT and the SSC guidelines, it is still important to remember the ABCDE approach to an acutely ill patient with severe sepsis. The key priority is early effective intervention which has been shown to improve outcome. Fig. 6.10 summarises the early management of severe sepsis.

> ### Key points: sepsis
> - Sepsis is a defined and important condition.
> - It is characterised by an over-response to infection, with uncontrolled inflammation, coagulation and disruption of the microcirculation leading to tissue hypoxia.
> - The Surviving Sepsis Campaign is an international collaboration to improve the diagnosis, management and treatment of sepsis.
> - Early goal directed therapy in sepsis improves outcome.
> - Invasive monitoring should be instituted early in severe sepsis to guide the administration of fluids and vaso-active drugs.
> - Severe sepsis is an ICU disease.

Self-assessment: case histories

1 A 29-year-old woman is brought to the emergency department drowsy with the following vital signs: BP 80/50 mmHg, pulse 130/min, RR 28/min, SpO$_2$ 95% on 10 l/min via reservoir bag mask and temperature 38.5°C. Her arterial blood gases show: pH 7.3, PaO$_2$ 35.5 (273 mmHg), PaCO$_2$ 3.5 (26.9 mmHg), st bicarbonate 12.7 mmol/l and BE -10. She has a purpuric rash on her trunk. She responds to voice, her bedside glucose measurement is 6.2 mmol/l (103 mg/dl) and there is no neck stiffness. What is your management?

2 A 40-year-old man is admitted with community acquired pneumonia and is started on appropriate i.v. antibiotics. Twenty four hours later you are asked to review him because he appears unwell. On examination he is alert, RR is 36/min, SpO$_2$ is 94% on 15 l/min via reservoir bag mask, BP is 130/70 mmHg and pulse is 105/min. He has a temperature of 38°C. His arterial blood gases show pH 7.3, PaO$_2$ 21 (161 mmHg), PaCO$_2$ 3.5 (26.9 mmHg), st bicarbonate 12.7 mmol/l and BE -10. What is your management?

3 A 52-year-old man has an emergency laparotomy for perforation of the colon following an elective colonoscopy. Twelve hours following surgery, his vital

signs are as follows: temperature 38°C, pulse 110/min, RR 30/min, BP 90/50 mmHg and poor urine output. He is mildly confused. Investigations show: Hb 10.5 g/dl, WBC 20×10^9/l, platelets 70×10^9/l, Na 135 mmol/l, K 4.7 mmol/l, urea 15 mmol/l (blood urea nitrogen (BUN) 41.6 mg/dl) and creatinine 150 μmol/l (1.8 mg/dl). Arterial blood gases on 5 l/min via Hudson mask show: pH 7.26, PO_2 8.2 (63 mmHg), PCO_2 5.3 (40.7 mmHg), st bicarbonate 17.5 mmol/l and BE −8. A CVP line has been inserted after 1500 ml colloid. The initial reading is 12 mmHg. What is your further management?

4 A 60-year-old woman was seen in the emergency department and treated for a urinary tract infection on the basis of symptoms and a positive urine dipstick. The next day she returns having collapsed. On arrival her observations are as follows: alert, pulse 120/min, temperature 39°C, BP 80/50 mmHg, RR 20/min, SpO_2 95% on air and urine output normal. What is your management?

5 A 19-year-old i.v. drug user is admitted at 3 AM with a severe hand infection due to injecting with dirty needles. His hand and arm are becoming increasingly swollen. He is alert but his other observations are: BP 70/40 mmHg, temperature 39°C, RR 24/min, SpO_2 95% on air and pulse 130/min. He has no peripheral venous access so the admitting junior doctor has prescribed high-dose oral antibiotics and decided to 'review him in the morning'. Describe your management.

6 A 45-year-old woman with severe rheumatoid arthritis is admitted with a painful right hip. She is on monthly infusions of Infliximab (an immunosuppressant drug) for her rheumatoid disease as well as daily steroids. Her admission blood tests show a raised C-reactive protein and neutrophil count. Her vital signs on admission are: BP 130/60 mmHg, temperature 36.7°C, RR 16/min, SpO_2 98% on air and pulse 80/min. She is alert. Twenty four hours later she develops hypotension (BP 75/40 mmHg) and a tachycardia (110/min). A blood culture report is phoned through as 'Staphylococcus aureus in both bottles'. She is alert, apyrexial, with a respiratory rate of 24/min, bilateral basal crackles (new) and SpO_2 of 87% on air. What is your management?

7 A 40-year-old man is admitted with abdominal pain which is diagnosed as acute pancreatitis (amylase of 2000 U/l). He is given high-concentration oxygen, i.v. fluids and analgesia. Six hours later he develops a poor urine output. His vital signs are: BP 95/60 mmHg, pulse 120/min, RR 25/min, SpO_2 90% on 10 l/min via reservoir bag mask, temperature 38°C and he is alert. Blood lactate is 4.5 mmol/l (normal 0.5–2.0 mmol/l). What is your management?

8 A 50-year-old man is admitted with a severe gastrointestinal bleed and receives 14 U of packed red cells plus other colloids during 4 h of stabilisation followed by upper gastrointestinal endoscopy. He is then transferred to theatre for surgical repair of a large bleeding duodenal ulcer. Twenty four hours after surgery he is still ventilated and has increasing oxygen requirements. A chest X-ray shows bilateral patchy infiltrates. His vital signs are: BP 110/70 mmHg, pulse 110/min, RR 14/min (ventilated), SpO_2 92% on

60% oxygen and temperature 37°C. What is the diagnosis and what is the management?

Self-assessment: discussion

1 This patient has severe sepsis, as defined in Fig. 6.2, and the purpuric rash is a pointer to meningococcal sepsis (although other infections can cause this). Severe sepsis is a serious condition – call for senior help now. Management starts with A (airway and high-concentration oxygen therapy), B (breathing) and C (circulation). Blood should be sent for full blood count, urea and electrolytes, liver tests, clotting and two sets of cultures. Lactate can be measured either by the lab urgently or by an arterial blood gas machine. Fluid boluses should be given to correct hypotension and hypoperfusion. Broad-spectrum antibiotics should be administered (2 g i.v. cefotaxime qds) [27]. Meningococcal disease evolves rapidly, so even if the patient responds to fluid boluses, she should be admitted to an ICU. A metabolic acidosis or hypotension should be treated with EGDT. Control hyperglycaemia if present. If vasopressors are required, give i.v. hydrocortisone. Patients with meningococcal sepsis have at least moderate coagulopathy and would therefore have been excluded from the PROWESS study [18]. Although these patients may benefit from the Drotrecogin Alfa (Activated), they are almost certainly at higher than usual risk of bleeding and a cautious approach is advised.

2 This patient also has severe sepsis, as defined in Fig. 6.2. Notice that there is evidence of hypoperfusion with a normal BP. Management starts with A (airway and high-concentration oxygen therapy), B (breathing, e.g. wheeze) and C (circulation). Blood should be sent as in case 1 and fluid boluses given to correct the metabolic acidosis. Other causes of metabolic acidosis should be screened for on examination and testing. The patient may respond to aggressive fluid resuscitation, and may simply require close monitoring of vital signs, respiratory function and lactate levels. If there is persisting hypoperfusion, he would benefit from more invasive monitoring and EGDT.

3 This patient has severe sepsis, caused by bacterial peritonitis. He requires high concentration oxygen and fluid boluses. Blood tests should be sent as in case 1 and appropriate antibiotics given, if not already. In this case, there is a persisting metabolic acidosis with hypotension despite a (probably) normal intravascular volume. Already, four organ systems are compromised, not including the gut: cardiovascular (hypotension), renal (poor urine output and raised creatinine), respiratory (hypoxaemia and normal $PaCO_2$ despite metabolic acidosis) and haematological (low platelets). Mortality associated with perforation varies according to site – <5% for small bowel and appendix, 10% for the gastro-duodenal tract, 20–30% for the colon and 50% for post-operative anastomotic leaks. Immediate referral to intensive care is required.

4 This patient has severe sepsis, caused by a urinary tract infection. High-concentration oxygen should be given despite her normal SpO_2. This is the

first step in maximising oxygen delivery to the tissues. Blood should be sent as in case 1, a urine sample should be obtained for culture and broad-spectrum i.v. antibiotics given (e.g. cefuroxime). Fluid boluses should be given. Arterial blood gases should be measured in any patient with severe sepsis to assess the degree of any metabolic (lactic) acidosis. If her hypotension and/or metabolic acidosis persists despite oxygen and fluid therapy, she requires more invasive monitoring and EGDT, as outlined in Figs 6.5 and 6.10.

5 This patient also has severe sepsis, but young patients who are alert can deceive inexperienced doctors into thinking the situation is not serious. Follow the algorithm in Fig. 6.10 (first step – call for senior help now). In this case, also worry about necrotising fasciitis (suggested by rapid progression, severe systemic upset and soft tissue crepitus) and developing compartment syndrome with rhabdomyolysis.

6 This patient has severe sepsis, caused by septic arthritis, and is also developing ALI (non-cardiogenic pulmonary oedema). This case illustrates how immunosuppressed patients do not necessarily get a fever. High-concentration oxygen is required, blood should be sent as in case 1 (including further cultures) and a fluid bolus administered. Give appropriate i.v. antibiotics (e.g. high-dose flucloxacillin pending further advice from the microbiology lab). Arterial blood gas analysis is required to assess oxygenation, ventilation and perfusion (ABC). Early invasive monitoring is required in this case as the patient is already developing signs of pulmonary oedema, which is likely to be exacerbated by fluid therapy. Contact the ICU team immediately.

7 This patient has SIRS caused by acute pancreatitis. The pathophysiological and clinical features are identical to severe sepsis. Management is pretty much the same as in Fig. 6.10, except that APC is used only in sepsis. Antibiotics are not necessarily given in SIRS (see case 8).

8 This patient probably also has SIRS (he is ventilated), caused by a massive blood transfusion and surgery. The predominant feature is ALI/ARDS. He is hypoxaemic despite a high FiO_2. He still requires optimisation of oxygen delivery and control of blood glucose. He should be ventilated in accordance with the recommendations for patients with ARDS.

References

1. Martin G, Mannino DM, Eaton S and Moss M. The epidemiology of sepsis in the United States from 1979 through 2000. *New England Journal of Medicine* 2003; **348**: 1546–1554.
2. Angus DC, Linde-Zwirble WT, Lidicker J, Clermont G, Carcillo J and Pinsky MR. Epidemiology of severe sepsis in the United States: analysis of incidence, outcome, and associated costs of care. *Critical Care Medicine* 2001; **29(7)**: 1303–1310.
3. Moreno R, Vincent JL, Matos R, Mendonca Q *et al*. The use of maximum SOFA scores to quantify organ dysfunction/failure in intensive care. Results of a prospective multicentre study. *Intensive Care Medicine* 1999; **25**: 686–696.
4. Members of the American College of Chest Physicians/Society of Critical Care Med consensus conference. Definitions for sepsis and organ failure and guidelines for the use of innovative therapies in sepsis. *Critical Care Medicine* 1992; **20**: 864–874.

5. Levy MM, Mitchell PF, Marshall JC *et al.* 2001 SCCM/ESICM/ACCP/ATS/SIS international sepsis definitions conference. *Critical Care Medicine* 2003; **31(4)**: 1250–1256.

6. www.sepsis.com. An educational resource for clinicians.

7. www.survivingsepsis.org

8. Dellinger RP, Carlet J, Masur H *et al.* Surviving sepsis campaign guidelines for the management of severe sepsis and septic shock. *Critical Care Medicine* 2004; **32(3)**: 858–872.

9. www.ihi.org/IHI/Topics/CriticalCare/Sepsis. The USA Institute for Healthcare Improvement website.

10. Smith I, Kumar P, Molloy S, Rhodes A *et al.* Base excess and lactate as prognostic indicators for patients admitted to intensive care. *Intensive Care Medicine* 2001; **27**: 74–83.

11. Bor DH and Aronson MD. Blood cultures: clinical decisions. In: Sox Jr HC, ed. *Common Diagnostic Tests.* American College of Physicians, Philadelphia, 1990.

12. Ibrahim EH, Sherman G, Ward S *et al.* The influence of inadequate microbial treatment of bloodstream infections on patient outcome in the ICU setting. *Chest* 2000; **118**: 146–155.

13. Fink M. Cytopathic hypoxia in sepsis. *Acta Anaesthesiologica Scandinavia Supplement* 1997; **110**: 87–95.

14. Rivers E, Nguyen B, Havstad S *et al.* Early goal-directed therapy in the treatment of severe sepsis and septic shock. *New England Journal of Medicine* 2001; **345(19)**: 1368–1377. Free limited registration at www.nejm.org allows access to this paper.

15. Gattinoni L, Brazzi L, Pelosi P *et al.* A trial of goal-oriented haemodynamic therapy in critically ill patients. *New England Journal of Medicine* 1995; **333**: 1025–1032.

16. Van den Berghe G, Wouters P, Weekers F *et al.* Intensive insulin therapy in the critically ill patient. *New England Journal of Medicine* 2001; **345**: 1359–1367.

17. Annane D, Bellissant E, Bollaert PE *et al.* Corticosteroids for treating severe sepsis and septic shock. *Cochrane Database Systematic Review* 2005; **1**: CD002243.

18. Bernard GR, Vincent JL, Laterre PF *et al.* Efficacy and safety of recombinant human activated protein C for severe sepsis. *New England Journal of Medicine* 2001; **344**: 699–709.

19. Bernard GR, Margolis BD, Shanies HM *et al.* Extended evaluation of recombinant human activated protein C United States Trial (ENHANCE US): a single-arm, phase 3B, multicenter study of Drotrecogin Alfa (Activated) in severe sepsis. *Chest* 2004; **125(6)**: 2206–2216.

20. Abraham E, Laterre P-F, Garg R *et al.* Drotregin Alfa (Activated) for adults with severe sepsis and low risk of death. *New England Journal of Medicine* 2005; **353**: 1332–1341.

21. Albanese J, Leone M and Garnier F. Renal effects of norepinephrine in septic and non septic patients. *Chest* 2004; **126**: 534–539.

22. Marik P and Mohedin M. The contrasting effects of dopamine and norepinephrine on systemic and splanchnic oxygen ulitisation in hyperdynamic sepsis. *Journal of American Medical Association* 1994; **272(17)**: 1354–1357.

23. Martin C, Viviand X, Leone M and Thirion X. Effect of norepinephrine on the outcome of septic shock. *Critical Care Medicine* 2000; **28**: 2758–2765.

24. Martin C, Papazian L, Perrin G *et al.* Norepinephrine or dopamine for treatment of hyperdynamic septic shock. *Chest* 1993; **103**: 1826–1831.

25. Bernard GR, Artigas A, Brigham KL *et al.* The American–European Consensus Conference on ARDS. *American Journal of Respiratory Critical Care Medicine* 1994; **149**: 818–824.

26. The Acute Respiratory Distress Syndrome Network. Ventilation with lower tidal volumes as compared with traditional tidal volumes for acute lung injury and the acute respiratory distress syndrome. *New England Journal of Medicine* 2000; **342**: 1301–1308.

27. www.britishinfectionsociety.org/meningitis.html. UK guidelines on the management of meningococcal meningitis or sepsis from the British Infection Society.

CHAPTER 7
Acute renal failure

By the end of this chapter you will be able to:

- Define acute renal failure (ARF)
- Know the factors which affect renal perfusion
- Know the common causes of ARF
- Appreciate the importance of preventing ARF
- Use a simple system for treating ARF
- Understand the principles of renal replacement therapy
- Apply this to your clinical practice

Definitions

Acute renal failure (ARF) has been defined in many different ways, but for practical purposes ARF is:

- A rapid (hours to weeks) decline in glomerular filtration rate (GFR) indicated by a rising creatinine
- With or without the development of oliguria (a urine output of less than 400 ml/day).

In catheterised patients, oliguria is also defined as a urine output of less than 0.5 ml/kg/h for two consecutive hours. Although arbitrary, a urine output below this figure is an important marker of renal hypoperfusion which should trigger assessment and action. However, up to half of the cases of ARF are non-oliguric. Anuria (0–100 ml/day) suggests obstruction until proven otherwise.

Urine output and creatinine are helpful, but are not accurate measures of renal function. Creatinine clearance is better and can be estimated by the equation:

$$\text{Clearance} = \frac{(140 - \text{age}) \times \text{weight in kg}}{\text{creatinine in } \mu\text{mol/l}} \quad (\times 1.2 \text{ for men})$$

For example, a normal creatinine can be deceptive in the elderly, who have less muscle mass. If an 80-year-old man weighing 60 kg has a creatinine of 100 μmol/l (1.2 mg/dl), his creatinine clearance is 43 ml/min, less than half of normal (around 100 ml/min), even though his creatinine is within the quoted normal range. The creatinine clearance calculation is often used for drug administration.

Renal perfusion

To understand why ARF happens, you need to first understand some basic renal physiology. Renal blood flow is normally 1200 ml/min, just over 20% cardiac output, one of the most highly perfused organs in the body. Various factors affect renal blood flow, as shown in Fig. 7.1.

There is autoregulation of renal blood flow between a mean arterial pressure of 70–170 mmHg in normal people. That is, the renal vascular bed adjusts in order to keep renal blood flow the same between these pressures:

$$\text{Renal blood flow} = \frac{\text{input pressure} - \text{output pressure}}{\text{resistance of renal vascular bed}}$$

Below a mean arterial pressure of 70 mmHg, autoregulation is no longer effective and both renal blood flow and GFR fall sharply. Autoregulation in hypertensive patients is shifted to the right, as shown in Fig. 7.2. This fact is

Renal vasoconstrictors	Renal vasodilators
Volume depletion	Atrial natriuretic peptide
Low mean arterial pressure	Nitric oxide
Sympathetic stimulation	Prostaglandins*
Increased angiotensin II levels	
Endothelin	

Figure 7.1 Factors affecting renal blood flow. *Increase cortical flow and reduce medullary flow.

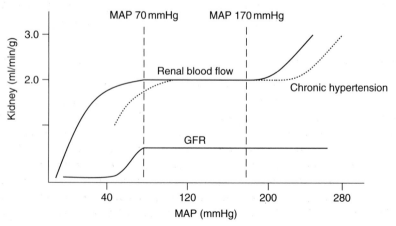

Figure 7.2 Renal blood flow. The renal blood flow autoregulation curve is shifted to the right in chronic hypertension.

important when treating normally hypertensive patients with ARF, as they may require a higher mean arterial pressure. The kidney is one of the vital organs in the body which depends on a critical *pressure* in order to function.

In other organs as blood flow falls, oxygen extraction increases to compensate. But in the kidney, oxygen uptake by the cells falls in parallel with blood flow. Initially the afferent (input) vessels dilate and the efferent (output) vessels constrict, to try and maintain an effective perfusion pressure in order to produce a glomerular filtrate. Total renal oxygen consumption is low except in the outer medulla where active sodium reabsorption occurs. This area is normally relatively hypoxic because of high tubular reabsorptive activity and is therefore particularly vulnerable to injury (acute tubular necrosis). Fig. 7.3 illustrates a nephron and some clinically important factors which affect its function at different sites.

Causes of ARF

Even though there are many causes of ARF, a reduction in renal blood flow leading to a reduced GFR represents the pathological final common pathway. Traditionally, causes of ARF are divided into three anatomical groups:

1 Pre-renal (volume depletion, reduced cardiac output, redistribution of blood flow, e.g. sepsis, liver failure)
2 Renal (acute tubular necrosis, vasculitis, emboli, glomerulonephritis, myeloma)
3 Post-renal (obstruction by prostrate, tumour or stones).

Pre-renal failure and acute tubular necrosis are the most common causes of ARF. Acute tubular necrosis is caused by any prolonged pre-renal cause, as well as toxins (e.g. drugs and contrast media). Sixty percent of community-acquired ARF is pre-renal [1]. In hospital-acquired ARF, renal hypoperfusion is the most common cause. However, 50% of hospital-acquired ARF is also multifactorial (e.g. sepsis treated with gentamicin in a patient with pre-existing renal impairment) [2]. Generally speaking, the causes of ARF do not vary with age, except that in the elderly, obstruction (post-renal failure) is more common [3].

Preventing ARF

Once established, ARF has a high mortality, 45% in one study [1]. Mortality is higher in males and in acute myocardial infarction, stroke, oliguria, sepsis and mechanical ventilation [4]. The kidney is especially vulnerable to injury resulting from hypoperfusion and/or critical illness. One prospective study looked at 2262 consecutive admissions to hospital to determine the contribution of iatrogenic factors in the development of ARF [5]. Patients admitted because of renal failure were excluded. The study found that 5% of hospital in-patients developed ARF. Despite the multitude of causes of ARF, a relatively small number of clinical scenarios accounted for the vast majority of hospital-acquired ARF:

• Hypoperfusion 42% (of these hypotension 41%, major cardiac dysfunction 30% and sepsis 19%)

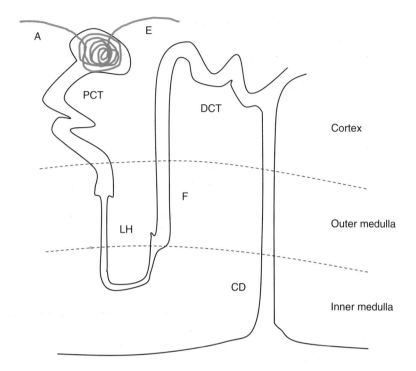

A: afferent arteriole where NSAIDs act, causing vasoconstriction. There is selective afferent vasodilatation by prostaglandins.

E: efferent arteriole where ACE inhibitors and angiotensin II blockers act, causing vasodilatation. There is selective efferent vasoconstriction by angiotensin II. In a person on an angiotensin converting enzyme (ACE) inhibitor and non-steroidal anti-inflammatory drug (NSAID) who is admitted with any condition causing hypovolaemia, both these drugs should be temporarily stopped. The combination of hypovolaemia and the action of these drugs dramatically reduces GFR. In cirrhosis and congestive cardiac failure where prostaglandins are recruited to increase renal blood flow, the renal effects of NSAIDs are even more potent.

F: thick ascending limb of the loop of Henle where frusemide blocks active sodium-potassium-chloride co-transport. Despite documented protective effects in experiments, frusemide has failed to prevent post-operative renal failure in high-risk patients or ameliorate established acute renal failure in clinical practice.

Figure 7.3 The nephron: functional unit of the kidney. PCT: proximal convoluted tubule; LH: thick and thin descending and ascending Loop of Henle; DCT: distal convoluted tubule; CD: collecting duct.

- Major surgery 18%
- Contrast media 12%
- Aminoglycoside administration 7%
- Miscellaneous 21% (e.g. obstruction, hepatorenal syndrome).

The severity of renal failure as indicated by the serum creatinine was the most important indicator of a poor prognosis.

From this and other research we know that certain patients are at risk of developing ARF in hospital [6]. These are patients with:

- Poor renal perfusion pressure (volume depletion, low cardiac output, diuretic therapy)
- Pre-existing renal impairment
- Diabetes
- Sepsis
- Vascular disease
- Liver disease.

It has been estimated that 55% of episodes of ARF in hospital are potentially avoidable as a result of fluid and drug mismanagement [5]. We know from the evidence presented in Chapter 1 that hypoperfusion is often treated suboptimally. Just like cardiac arrest, with its high mortality, ARF can be prevented in many cases by close monitoring of at risk patients and prompt intervention when things start to go wrong.

Pathophysiology of ARF

The pathophysiology behind ARF is complex and only partly understood. Much data comes from animal models where acute tubular necrosis is induced by transiently clamping a renal artery. Real patients are more complex, where renal failure is often part of a developing multi-system illness. As mentioned, the outer renal medulla is relatively hypoxic and prone to injury. When there is an ischaemic or septic insult, inflammatory mediators damage the endothelium.

Acute tubular necrosis is not as simple as damaged tubular cells sloughing and blocking the collecting ducts; there is a complex response which involves programmed cell death (apoptosis) and damage to the actin cytoskeleton which facilitates cell to cell adhesion and forms the barrier between blood and filtrate. Genetic factors also play a role. 'Knockout' mice without the gene for a cell adhesion molecule ICAM-1 (which helps leucocytes bind to the endothelium) do not develop ARF after an ischaemic insult [7].

In animal models, interruption of blood flow for less than 25 min results in oliguria but no anatomical changes and renal function returns to normal; 60–120 min of interrupted blood flow causes tubular cell damage (the metabolically active cells), but renal recovery is possible if further insults are avoided. Interruption of blood blow for longer than 120 min causes renal infarction and irreversible ARF. High-risk surgical procedures for the development of ARF are cardiac surgery, vascular surgery, urological surgery and procedures or conditions associated with intra-abdominal hypertension. Biliary and hepatic conditions also pose a risk because bile salts bind endotoxins which cause renal vasoconstriction and this action ceases in cholestasis.

Recovery from ARF does not only depend on restoration of renal blood flow, although this is obviously important. In intrinsic renal failure, once renal blood flow is restored, the remaining functional nephrons increase their filtration and hypertrophy. Recovery is dependent on the number of remaining functional nephrons. If this is below a critical value, continued hyperfiltration results in progressive glomerular sclerosis, which eventually leads to nephron loss. Continued nephron loss causes more hyperfiltration until renal failure results. This has been termed the hyperfiltration theory of renal failure and explains why progressive renal failure is sometimes observed after apparent recovery from ARF [7].

How to manage ARF

Early action saves kidneys. A simple system for managing ARF involves five steps:
1 Treat hyperkalaemia if present (see Box 7.1)
2 Correct hypovolaemia and establish an effective circulating volume
3 Treat hypoperfusion
4 Exclude obstruction
5 Stop nephrotoxins and treat the underlying cause (involve an expert).
The history, observations and drug chart usually reveal the cause of ARF. Life-threatening hyperkalaemia (above 6.5 mmol/l) should be treated first. The next step is to treat hypovolaemia (discussed in Chapter 5). After that, some patients may be euvolaemic but still have a blood pressure too low to adequately perfuse their kidneys (e.g. in severe sepsis or cardiogenic shock). Antihypertensive medication should be stopped and consideration should be given to the use of vaso-active drugs. A sample of urine should be sent for analysis and the patient catheterised in order to accurately measure urine output. Ideally a urine sample should be obtained before catheterisation as

---

Box 7.1 Treatment of hyperkalaemia

- Double-check with the laboratory that the sample was not haemolysed.
- Attach a cardiac monitor to the patient.
- Give 10 ml of 10% calcium chloride i.v. (slow bolus) for cardiac protection.
- Give 50 ml of 50% dextrose i.v. (10 U of actrapid insulin is added if the patient is unlikely to mount an adequate insulin response). Monitor capillary glucose measurements.
- Check serum K^+ 1-h later.
- If serum K^+ still high, give another 50 ml of 50% dextrose i.v.
- If serum K^+ still high, give 100 ml of 4.2% sodium bicarbonate i.v.
- Salbutamol nebulisers can also be added.
- Stop food and drugs that cause hyperkalaemia.
- Calcium resonium can be added for longer-term prevention.

this procedure can cause microscopic haematuria. An urgent renal tract ultra-sound should be arranged to look for obstruction. Finally, it is important to stop all nephrotoxic drugs and treat the underlying cause of ARF. A list of common nephrotoxic drugs is shown in Fig. 7.4.

Urinalysis is an important test in the evaluation of ARF, not least because urinary tract infection is an important cause of ARF, especially in the elderly (see Fig. 7.5). Urinalysis can also point towards more unusual causes of ARF, such as glomerulonephritis (proteinuria, red cells, casts).

Although glomerulonephritis causes less than 5% of ARF, it is an important diagnosis which should not be overlooked. Fortunately, acute glomerulonephritis as a cause of ARF is rarely subtle [8]. Urinalysis is abnormal, constitutional symptoms are common and a rash is frequently seen. If the cause of the ARF

- ACE inhibitors
- Angiotensin II receptor antagonists (the 'sartans')
- NSAIDs
- Cox 2 inhibitors
- Diuretics
- Aminoglycosides
- Lithium
- A wide range of antibiotics
- Tacrolimus and cyclosporin (used in organ transplant patients)
- Amphoteracin B

The British National Formulary (BNF) section on renal impairment should be checked before prescribing any drug for a patient with acute renal failure.

Figure 7.4 Common nephrotoxic drugs.

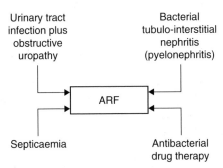

Figure 7.5 ARF caused by urinary tract infection. There is evidence to suggest a direct effect on the kidney by endotoxins. Dehydration due to vomiting also contributes. © A Raine, 1992. Reprinted from Advanced Renal Medicine by AEG Raine (1992) by permission of Oxford University Press.

is unclear, or if there are features to suggest a systemic disorder such as lupus, vasculitis, or a pulmonary-renal syndrome, contact a renal physician urgently.

There are various urine electrolyte tests that can help diagnose renal or pre-renal causes of ARF. These are based on the fact that in pre-renal failure the kidney avidly reabsorbs salt and water, but in intrinsic renal failure tubular function is disrupted and the kidney loses sodium in the urine. However, diuretic use increases the urinary excretion of sodium, making urinary sodium values difficult to interpret and these tests are rarely helpful in the majority of patients for whom there is a clear precipitating cause for their ARF.

Many cases of ARF respond to treatment using the five steps above. But what happens next if your patient continues to have a rising creatinine despite these measures? If the patient remains oliguric, frusemide can be used to treat fluid overload. Renal replacement therapy (RRT) is the next step and is required in approximately one third of patients [9], but only a small percentage require long-term dialysis [1].

Many treatments improve urine output but have no effect on outcome in established ARF:
• High dose loop diuretics (bolus or infusion)
• Mannitol
• Dopamine.

Frusemide is said to cause a reduction in renal oxygen demand and mannitol is thought to scavenge free radicals – theoretical benefits which are not borne out in clinical practice. However, loop diuretics can convert oliguric renal failure to non-oliguric renal failure and thus avoid problems with fluid overload. Diuretic resistance occurs in renal failure (and congestive cardiac failure) because of reduced diuretic delivery to the urine and a reduced natriuretic response. High doses or continuous infusions may therefore be required.

Renal replacement therapy: haemodialysis and haemofiltration

The indications for renal replacement therapy (RRT) in ARF are as follows [11]:
• Resistant hyperkalaemia
• Volume overload unresponsive to loop diuretics
• Worsening severe metabolic acidosis
• Uraemic complications (e.g. encephalopathy, pericarditis and seizures).

Haemodialysis

Haemodialysis removes solutes from blood by their passage across a semi-permeable membrane. Heparinised blood flows in one direction and dialysis fluid flows in another at a faster rate. Dialysis fluid contains physiological levels of electrolytes except potassium, which is low, and molecules cross the membrane by simple diffusion along a concentration gradient. Smaller molecules

Mini-tutorial: rhabdomyolysis

In certain situations, diuretics are used early in ARF, after restoration of intravascular volume. These are rhabdomyolysis and poisoning (e.g. lithium, theophylline and salicylates). Rhabdomyolysis is an important cause of ARF. It occurs when there is massive breakdown of muscle. Myoglobin is released into the circulation along with other toxins which leads to kidney dysfunction and general metabolic upset. Unlike many other causes of ARF, prognosis is good in rhabdomyolysis and the kidneys usually recover. Causes of rhabdomyolysis include:
• Crush injury/reperfusion after compartment syndrome
• Prolonged immobility following a fall or overdose, especially with hypothermia
• Drug overdose (e.g. ecstasy, carbon monoxide poisoning)
• Extreme exertion
• Myositis (caused by influenza, severe hypokalaemia or drugs like statins)
• Malignant hyperthermia (triggered by some anaesthetic agents)
• Neuroleptic malignant syndrome

Myoglobin and urate from muscle breakdown are said to obstruct the tubules. Yet tubular obstruction is probably not what causes ARF in rhabdomyolysis, because studies show that intratubular pressures are normal. More likely is free-radical-mediated injury. Renal vasoconstriction also occurs, partly because of the underlying cause and partly because myoglobin itself causes vasoconstriction [10].

The typical blood picture in rhabdomyolysis is a high creatinine, potassium and phosphate, low calcium and a creatinine kinase (CK) in the tens of thousands. Fluid resuscitation remains the most important aspect of management in rhabdomyolysis. Early and aggressive i.v. fluid has dramatic benefits on outcome when compared to historical controls. Guidelines go as far as 12 l of fluid a day to 'flush' the kidneys and achieve a urine output of 200–300 ml/h [10]. Alkalinisation of the urine significantly improves renal function, probably by inhibiting free-radical-mediated damage. The urine is dipsticked every hour and sodium bicarbonate is given i.v. to raise the urine pH to 7.0. Mannitol is the first line diuretic in rhabdomyolysis, but its use in addition to fluid therapy has not been shown to be more effective than fluid therapy alone. Frusemide acidifies the urine but is sometimes administered after a trial of mannitol. Plasmapheresis is not an established therapy in rhabdomyolysis, although myoglobin can be removed from the circulation this way.

move faster than larger ones. Urea and creatinine concentrations are zero in the dialysis fluid. A 3–4 h treatment can reduce urea by 70%. Water can be removed by applying a pressure gradient across the membrane if needed.

Haemofiltration

Haemofiltration involves blood under pressure moving down one side of a semi-permeable membrane. This has a similar effect to glomerular filtration and small and large molecules are cleared at the same rates. Instead of selective reabsorption, which occurs in the kidney, the whole filtrate is discarded and the

Component	Value (mmol/l)
Sodium	140
Potassium	4
Calcium	1.75
Magnesium	0.75
Chloride	109
Lactate	40
Glucose	11

Figure 7.6 Typical composition of haemofiltration replacement fluid.

patient is infused with a replacement physiological solution instead (see Fig. 7.6). Less fluid may be replaced than is removed in cases of fluid overload. In original haemofiltration, the femoral artery and vein were cannulated (continuous arteriovenous haemofiltration, CAVH). Blood passed through the filter under arterial pressure alone – but circuit disconnection could lead to rapid blood loss and patients with low blood pressures often had slow moving circuits with the associated risk of blood clotting. In more common use today is continuous veno-venous haemofiltration (CVVH). A large vein is cannulated using a double lumen catheter and a pump controls blood flow. The extracorporeal circuit is anticoagulated in both CAVH and CVVH. Automated systems have a replacement fluid pump which can either balance input and output or allow a programmed rate of fluid loss.

Haemofiltration removes virtually all ions from plasma including calcium and bicarbonate. Replacing these is difficult, since solutions containing enough of these two ions can precipitate. Lactate is commonly used instead of bicarbonate – but although in normal people lactate is converted to bicarbonate, this is not true of patients with lactic acidosis. In these situations bicarbonate infusions must be given separately. CVVH has advantages over haemodialysis in the critical care setting because it avoids the hypotension often seen in dialysis, can continuously remove large volumes of water in patients receiving parenteral nutrition and other infusions, offers better clearance of urea and solutes, may better preserve cerebral perfusion pressure and also has a role in clearing inflammatory mediators [12]. The difference between haemodialysis and haemofiltration is shown in Fig. 7.7.

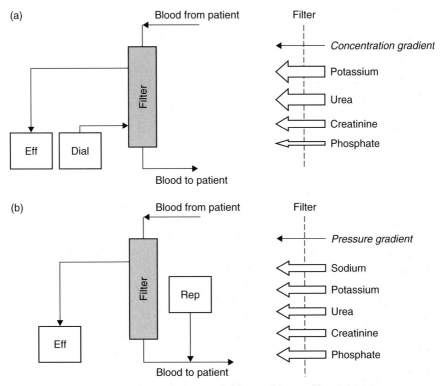

Figure 7.7 The difference between haemodialysis and haemofiltration. (a) Continuous veno-venous haemodialysis and (b) continuous veno-venous haemofiltration. Eff: effluent; Dial: dialysis fluid; Rep: replacement fluid.

Mini-tutorial: low dose dopamine for ARF

The use of low dose dopamine at 0.2–2.5 μg/kg/min (or 'renal dose') for ARF still occurs despite the fact that randomised trials have shown it is of no benefit either as prevention in high-risk post-operative patients or as treatment in established ARF [13]. The effects of a dopamine infusion are complicated because it acts on a number of different receptors which have opposing actions. The action of dopamine is not constant throughout its dose range. Stimulation of α-receptors causes systemic vasoconstriction and the blood pressure rises. β1-receptors increase contractility of the heart, β2-receptors reduce afterload and dopamine (DA) receptors cause renal and splanchnic vasodilatation. Dopamine acts on all these receptors. In addition, there are two major subgroups of dopamine receptor. DA1 receptors are in the renal and mesenteric circulation. DA2 receptors are in the autonomic ganglia and sympathetic nerve endings and inhibit noradrenaline release. Dopamine and its synthetic sister dopexamine have been used extensively to theoretically improve renal blood flow and therefore function. Dopexamine is also used to improve splanchnic blood flow in certain post-operative situations [14].

Dopamine causes a diuresis and natriuresis independent of any effect on renal blood flow by inhibiting proximal tubule Na–K–ATPase (via DA1 and DA2 stimulation). So the effect we see with low dose dopamine is a diuresis – not a change in creatinine clearance [15]. In one randomised prospective double-blind trial, 23 patients at risk for renal dysfunction were given either dopamine at 200 μg/min, dobutamine at 175 μg/min or 5% dextrose [16]. Dopamine increased urine output without a change in creatinine clearance and dobutamine caused a significant increase in creatinine clearance by increasing cardiac output without an increase in urine output. This illustrates the difficulty of using urine output as a surrogate marker for renal function.

Critically ill patients have reduced dopamine clearance and a wide variability in plasma dopamine levels. One cannot therefore assume that low dose dopamine is acting only on the renal circulation. Treatment with dopamine could lead to unwanted side effects such as tachyarrhythmias, increased afterload and reduced respiratory drive [15]. In summary, there is no evidence to justify the use of low dose dopamine in the treatment of ARF.

Key points: acute renal failure

- ARF is defined as a rapid rise in creatinine with or without oliguria.
- The kidneys rely on a critical pressure in order to function.
- Pre-renal factors most commonly cause ARF, although for hospital in-patients, it is often multifactorial.
- ARF can be prevented and at risk patients should be monitored closely.
- ARF should be treated early using five simple steps – once established, it carries a high mortality.
- Involve an expert if the cause of ARF is unclear, due to intrinsic renal pathology or the condition fails to respond to simple measures.

Self-assessment: case histories

1 A 30-year-old man was admitted after being found lying on the floor of his apartment. He had taken i.v. heroin the night before. His admission blood results show a normal full blood count, sodium 130 mmol/l, potassium 6 mmol/l, urea 64 mmol/l (blood urea nitrogen, BUN 177 mg/dl) and creatinine 500 μmol/l (6 mg/dl). His vital signs are: drowsy, blood pressure 90/60 mmHg, pulse 100/min, temperature 35°C, respiratory rate 8/min and oxygen saturations 95% on air. What is your management?

2 A 60-year-man is admitted with a general deterioration in health. He is treated for heart failure and is taking the following medications: ramipril 10 mg, frusemide 80 mg and allopurinol 300 mg at night. He had been treated for a chest infection and pleurisy a week before admission with amoxycillin and a non-steroidal anti-inflammatory drug (NSAID). On examination he is drowsy and appears dehydrated. His blood pressure is 70/40 mmHg,

gentamicin therapy and a previous nephrectomy – early action is essential to prevent irreversible damage to his remaining kidney. Persisting hypoperfusion despite adequate volume replacement would require vaso-active drugs in a Level 2–3 facility. Obstruction should be excluded. The underlying cause (common bile duct stone and cholangitis) should be treated as soon as possible.

5 The history and examination in this case point to volume depletion which should be corrected with fluid challenges. Note that she is known to have hypertension. What is her usual blood pressure? Follow the five steps in the management of ARF. The underlying cause in this case is likely to be dehydration and NSAID use.

6 The peri-operative period can be associated with episodes of hypoperfusion (because of volume depletion from many causes and hypotension due to anaesthesia). Peri-operative NSAID use can precipitate ARF, especially in the elderly. Stopping the NSAIDs and other nephrotoxins, and giving fluid may enough the reverse the ARF in this case.

7 This man was at risk of developing ARF because he had pre-existing diabetic renal disease and has had a major cardiovascular upset. A period of hypoperfusion has caused ARF. Management is the same as in the other cases: treat any life-threatening hyperkalaemia first, then hypovolaemia, then any hypoperfusion, catheterise, exclude higher obstruction with an ultrasound scan and treat the underlying cause. If renal function continues to deteriorate, RRT should be considered.

8 The patient is likely to be volume depleted as indicated by the history, examination and metabolic acidosis. The cross-clamping of the aorta also puts her at risk of developing ARF. She should be 'warmed up and filled up'. Rewarming causes vasodilatation which reveals pre-existing hypovolaemia. Dopexamine is often used in post-aneurysm repair patients because a few small studies have suggested a beneficial effect on creatinine clearance following major surgery – probably due to increased cardiac output and systemic vasodilatation. However, the vast majority of clinical studies of dopamine and dopexamine following major surgery have not demonstrated a benefit.

References

1. Liano F and Pascual J. Madrid Acute Renal Failure Study Group. Epidemiology of acute renal failure: a prospective, multi-center community based study. *Kidney International* 1996; **50**: 811–818.
2. Star RA. Treatment of acute renal failure. *Kidney International* 1998; **54**: 1817–1831.
3. Pascual J and Liano F. The Madrid Acute Renal Failure Study Group. Causes and prognosis of acute renal failure in the very old. *Journal of the American Geriatrics Society* 1998; **46**: 1–5.
4. Ball CM and Phillips RS. Acute renal failure. In: *Acute Medicine (Evidence-Based On-Call Series)*. Churchill Livingstone, London, 2001.

5. Hou SH, Bushinsky DA, Wish JB, Cohen JJ and Harrington JT. Hospital-acquired renal insufficiency: a prospective study. *American Journal of Medicine* 1993; **74**: 243–248.
6. Galley HF. Can acute renal failure be prevented? [educational review]. *Journal of the Royal College of Surgeons of Edinburgh* 2000; **45(1)**: 44–50.
7. Plant WD. Pathophysiology of acute renal failure. In: Galley HF, ed. *Renal Failure (Critical Care Focus Series)*. Intensive Care Society/BMJ Books, London, 1999.
8. Albright Jr RC. Acute renal failure: a practical update. *Mayo Clinic Proceedings* 2001; **76**: 67–74.
9. Thadhani R, Pascual M and Bonventre JV. Acute renal failure. *New England Journal of Medicine* 1996; **334**: 1448–1460.
10. Holt SG. Rhabdomyolysis. In: Galley HF, ed. *Renal Failure (Critical Care Focus Series)*. Intensive Care Society/BMJ Books, London, 1999.
11. Lameire N, Van Biesen W and Vanholder R. Acute renal failure. *Lancet* 2005; **365**: 417–430.
12. Forni LG and Hilton PJ. Continuous haemofiltration in the treatment of acute renal failure. *New England Journal of Medicine* 1997; **336**: 1303–1309.
13. Kellum JA and Decker JM. Use of dopamine in acute renal failure: a meta-analysis. *Critical Care Medicine* 2001; **29(8)**: 1526–1531.
14. Renton MC and Snowden CP. Dopexamine and its role in the protection of hepatosplanchnic and renal perfusion in high-risk surgical and critically ill patients. *British Journal of Anaesthesia* 2005; **94(4)**: 459–467.
15. Burton CJ and Tomson CRV. Can the use of low-dose dopamine for treatment of acute renal failure be justified? *Postgraduate Medical Journal* 1999; **75(883)**: 269–274.
16. Duke GJ, Briedis JH and Weaver RA. Renal support in critically ill patients: low dose dopamine or low dose dobutamine? *Critical Care Medicine* 1994; **22(12)**: 1919–1924.

Further resource

- www.kidneyatlas.org/toc.htm On-line chapters from Atlas of Diseases of the Kidney.

CHAPTER 8
Brain failure

By the end of this chapter you will be able to:

- Understand some of the basic physiology of the brain
- Know the difference between primary and secondary brain injury
- Be able to apply the principles of brain protection
- Manage an unconscious patient
- Know the prognosis following cardiac arrest
- Apply this to your clinical practice

The previous chapters have related to A (airway/oxygen), B (breathing) and C (circulation). This chapter is about D (disability) and concentrates on two important themes in the management of an acutely ill patient: brain protection and the unconscious patient. But first you need to understand some basic brain physiology.

Cerebral blood flow

Cerebral blood flow (CBF) is around 15% of cardiac output and is affected by various factors. The main ones are as follows:

- $PaCO_2$: A high $PaCO_2$ causes vasodilatation of blood vessels and increases CBF. A low $PaCO_2$ causes vasoconstriction. Reducing the $PaCO_2$ from 5 to 4 kPa (38.5–30.5 mmHg) reduces CBF by almost 30%.
- Hypoxaemia: Below 6.7 kPa (51.5 mmHg) causes increasing CBF.
- Mean arterial pressure (MAP).
- Drugs.

The relationship of CBF to $PaCO_2$, PaO_2 and MAP is shown in Fig. 8.1.

Like the kidneys, the brain autoregulates blood flow so that it is constant between a MAP of 50 and 150 mmHg. CBF is regulated by changes in the resistance of the cerebral arteries. Unlike the rest of the body, the larger arteries play a main role in this autoregulation. Local chemicals, endothelial mediators and neurogenic factors are thought to be responsible.

CBF is controlled by alterations in cerebral perfusion pressure (CPP) and cerebral vascular resistance (R):

$$CBF = \frac{CPP}{R}$$

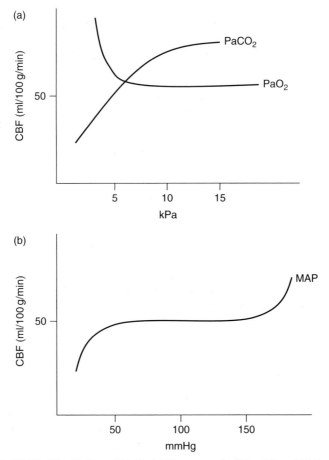

Figure 8.1 CBF, $PaCO_2$, PaO_2 and MAP. (a) Between a $PaCO_2$ of 2 and 9 kPa there is an almost linear increase in CBF. There is little change in CBF until below a PaO_2 of 6.7 kPa. (b) Autoregulation of cerebral perfusion occurs between MAP of 50 and 150. Beyond these limits, CBF is dramatically affected.

CPP is the pressure gradient in the brain or the difference between the incoming arteries and the outgoing veins:

CPP = MAP − venous pressure

Venous pressure is equal to intracranial pressure (ICP), so CPP is usually expressed as:

CPP = MAP − ICP

Normal supine ICP is 7–17 mmHg and is frequently measured on neuro-intensive care units (ICUs). CPP can then be calculated and manipulated.

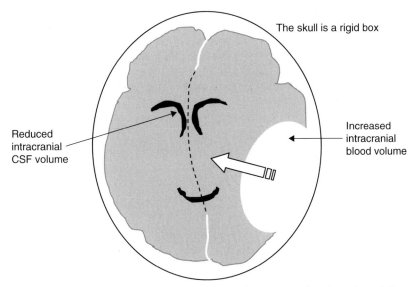

The skull is a rigid box

Reduced
intracranial
CSF volume

Increased
intracranial
blood volume

Figure 8.2 The Monro–Kellie doctrine. Diagram of a CT scan showing a large left extradural haematoma with midline shift.

Intracranial pressure

The skull is a rigid box and its contents are incompressible, therefore, ICP depends on the volume of intracranial contents: 5% blood, 10% cerebrospinal fluid (CSF) and 85% brain. The Monro–Kellie doctrine, named after two Scottish anatomists (see Fig. 8.2), states that as the cranial cavity is a closed box, any change in intracranial blood volume is accompanied by an opposite change in CSF volume, if ICP is to be maintained.

When ICP is raised the following occurs:

- CSF moves into the spinal canal and there is increased reabsorption into the venous circulation
- Compensatory mechanisms are eventually overwhelmed so further small changes in volume lead to large changes in pressure (see Fig. 8.3)
- As ICP rises further, CPP and CBF decrease
- Eventually brainstem herniation (coning) occurs.

The clinical features of acutely raised ICP are headache, nausea and vomiting, confusion, and a reduced conscious level. This can occur in traumatic brain injury, cerebral haemorrhage or infarction, meningitis/encephalitis, or quickly growing tumours. An estimate of ICP can be made in patients with brain injury who are not sedated:

- Drowsy and confused with Glasgow Coma Score (GCS) 13–15: ICP 20 mmHg
- GCS less than 8: ICP 30 mmHg.

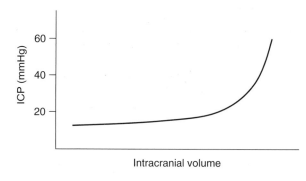

Figure 8.3 Effect of increasing intracranial volume on ICP.

Primary and secondary brain injury

Primary brain injury is the injury that has already occurred and has limited treatment. But the brain is uniquely vulnerable to *secondary* insults and less capable of maintaining an adequate blood flow and metabolic balance following injury. Research in the field of traumatic brain injury has shown that preventing secondary brain injury can improve outcome for the patient. Secondary brain injury is, by definition, delayed and therefore amenable to intervention. Examples of secondary brain injury include:
- Raised ICP
- Ischaemia
- Oedema
- Infection (e.g. in open fractures).

Following brain injury, neurones are rendered dysfunctional although not mechanically destroyed. If the subsequent environment is favourable, many of these cells can recover. Preventing raised ICP and saving the penumbra (the area around the primary injury with its compromised microcirculation) is important. An uncontrolled increase in ICP and brainstem herniation is the major cause of death after traumatic brain injury or intracerebral haemorrhage. In traumatic brain injury, the main precipitants of secondary injury are hypotension and hypoxaemia. Hypoxaemia, as defined by oxygen saturations <93%, and hypotension, as defined by a systolic BP of less than 90 mmHg, are associated with a statistically significant worse outcome and are common at the scene of injury [1].

Principles of brain protection

Based on our knowledge of brain physiology and observations of traumatic brain injury, a set of measures to protect the brain against secondary injury can be devised [2]. This can be applied to any kind of brain injury, for example, subarachnoid haemorrhage (SAH), meningitis or stroke.

Blood	CSF	Brain tissue
Avoid high $PaCO_2$ Avoid low PaO_2	Surgical drainage	Mannitol for generalised oedema
Nurse head up 15° if possible		Steroids for tumour-related oedema
Avoid coughing and straining		Frusemide is also sometimes used
Keep head in midline to facilitate venous drainage		

Figure 8.4 Methods to reduce ICP.

	Management
A	Secure airway (with cervical spine control in trauma)
	Treat hypoxaemia
B	Maintain normal $PaCO_2$
C	Treat hypotension (colloids give less interstitial volume increases)
	Maintain MAP at around 90 mmHg
D	Mannitol/steroids for oedema or surgery for evacuation of haematomas
	CSF shunt if indicated
	Treat fever
	Avoid placing patient head down
	Ensure adequate sedation and analgesia in intubated patients
E	Full neurological examination, investigations and planning

Figure 8.5 Summary of basic management to prevent secondary brain injury.

The aim of brain protection is to prevent:
- Raised ICP
- Cerebral ischaemia
- Cerebral oedema.

In addition, fever has been observed to worsen outcome in patients with brain injury, probably because the cerebral metabolic rate for oxygen is increased and this exacerbates local ischaemia.

Raised ICP is caused by an increase in the volume of blood, CSF or brain tissue, so treatment is aimed at reducing the volume of these three components and is summarised in Fig. 8.4.

Fig. 8.5 summarises these principles in an ABCDE format. Although most research has been done in traumatic brain injury, these principles have also been successfully applied to medical conditions such as meningitis with raised ICP [3], and current research is focussing on prevention of secondary brain injury in stroke.

Experimental methods of brain protection

The cerebral metabolic rate for oxygen is reduced by hypothermia. Hypothermia has been used in the past for cerebral protection during complex cardiac and neurosurgery. Animal models demonstrate its benefits but actively cooling normothermic human subjects with brain injury has not yet been shown to improve outcome [4]. However pyrexia is associated with an adverse outcome in brain injury [5] and therefore should be treated with paracetamol and active cooling.

Hypertonic saline has been studied extensively in traumatic brain injury. The theory is that the hypertonic solution will draw intracellular water into the intravascular space, reducing cerebral oedema and expanding intravascular volume. The results of clinical trials have been mixed [6]. In patients with other injuries such as haemorrhage or burns, resuscitation with hypertonic saline has adverse effects, so its use is not recommended in the routine resuscitation of trauma victims.

The unconscious patient

A reduced conscious level is associated with potentially life-threatening complications (e.g. airway obstruction and hypoxaemia, aspiration and immobilisation injuries) which require urgent intervention. Unconsciousness, or coma, is present when the GCS is 8 or less (see Fig. 8.6). Comatose patients should be referred to the ICU.

The causes of non-traumatic coma (lasting more than 6 h) are [7]:
• Sedative overdose: 40%
• Hypoxic brain injury: 24%
• Cerebrovascular disease: 18%

		Score
Eye opening	Spontaneous To speech To pain Nil	4 3 2 1
Best motor response	Obeys commands Localises pain Withdraws to pain Abnormal flexion to pain Extensor response to pain Nil	6 5 4 3 2 1
Best verbal response	Orientated Confused conversation Inappropriate words Incomprehensible sounds Nil	5 4 3 2 1

Figure 8.6 Glasgow Coma Score.

- Metabolic coma (e.g. infection, diabetes, hepatic encephalopathy, hypothermia): 15%
- Others: 3%.

However, a slightly different pattern is observed in the elderly, who commonly become confused, drowsy or unresponsive due to a wide range of conditions, most commonly infection and dehydration.

Seizures are an important, although less common, cause of coma, either because the patient is post-ictal (which can be prolonged in the elderly) or has non-convulsive status epilepticus [8].

A systematic approach is required in the management of an unconscious patient. As usual, the ABCDE system is used:

- A: assess and treat *airway* problems.
- B: assess and treat *breathing* problems.
- C: assess and treat *circulation* problems.
- D: assess *disability* (pupil size and reactivity, capillary glucose and the simple Alert, responds to Voice, responds to Pain, Unresponsive (AVPU) scale) and treat any problems. The GCS should be recorded once A, B and C are stable so that any later changes can be documented precisely.
- E: includes a full neurological *examination*. Certain clusters of signs may point to a particular diagnosis (see Fig. 8.7).

Deliberation and diagnosis must not take precedence over the assessment and treatment of ABC problems. For example, early antibiotic therapy in meningitis is crucial, however relieving airway obstruction and giving i.v. fluid for hypotension is just as important.

The indications for tracheal intubation in patients with brain injury are the same as in any other patient, that is GCS of 8 or less, airway problems and the need for ventilation, but in certain situations patients may need intubation

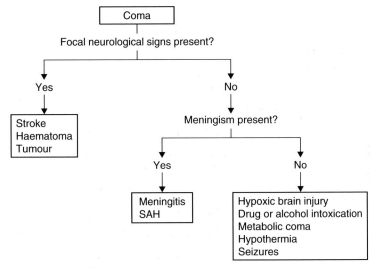

Figure 8.7 Clusters of signs in coma.

prior to transfer, for example, a deteriorating conscious level, bilateral mandible fractures, bleeding into the airway or seizures.

Imaging in coma

Computed tomography (CT) and magnetic resonance imaging (MRI) are the two techniques used in acutely ill adults. CT is the investigation of choice in trauma, subarachnoid haemorrhage (SAH) and stroke. It is readily available, quick and virtually all patients can be scanned. MRI provides images in several planes and provides superior grey/white matter contrast with a high sensitivity for most pathological processes compared with CT. MRI would be the investigation of choice in suspected posterior fossa lesions, seizures or inflammatory processes. MRI is also more sensitive for thin extradural haematomas and diffuse axonal injury in trauma but requires special consideration for anaesthetised patients because of the incompatibility of anaesthetic and monitoring equipment with the electromagnetic field.

Brain imaging is only undertaken if the patient is stable and a full evaluation has led to a differential diagnosis. When imaging is requested, it should lead to a diagnosis or have the potential to change management.

Mini-tutorial: subarachnoid haemorrhage

SAH is an uncommon cause of headache overall. However, if only patients presenting with the worst headache of their lives and a normal neurological examination are considered, SAH is more frequent, 12% in one study [9]. Neurological examination is often normal and in these cases one-third of patients are misdiagnosed. Delayed diagnosis leads to worse outcome. In one study 65% of misdiagnosed patients rebled [10].

SAH commonly presents with a thunderclap headache – a distinct, sudden, severe headache. It need not be in any location; neck pain or vomiting may predominate. The headache can resolve with painkillers. ECG changes commonly occur. The first episode of severe headache cannot be classified as migraine or tension headache (International Headache Society) [11]. Non-contrast CT scans are sensitive, but the pick-up rate decreases each day (92% on the same day, 76% 2 days later and 58% 5 days later) [12]. A negative CT scan does not exclude SAH.

Lumbar puncture (LP) should be performed to look for xanthochromia in cases with a suggestive history and negative CT scan. Although some authors have advocated waiting 12 h before LP [13] because xanthochromia takes time to form, others recommend immediate investigation [12]. SAH is also suggested by more than 1000 red cells/mm^3 but traumatic taps are common.

Patients with a SAH should be transferred to a neurosurgical unit as soon as possible for further assessment and management of their condition. Of patients with SAH who reach hospital, one-third will be in a coma, one-third will have neurological signs and one-third will make a good recovery. Interventional radiology techniques are now standard practice in the treatment of symptomatic intracranial aneurysms [14].

Prognosis following cardiac arrest

The incidence of sudden cardiac death is the same as the incidence of cancer in developed countries [15]. In most cases, outside hospital, it is due to ischaemic heart disease and ventricular fibrillation. Cardiac arrest and cardiopulmonary resuscitation (CPR) are commonly portrayed on television. Health care staff in popular US television dramas performed CPR in 62% of observed episodes and two-thirds of patients survived [16]. In reality, survival from out-of-hospital cardiac arrest is around 5–10% and many of these patients have neurological impairment [17–19]. However, studies have shown the effectiveness of rapid defibrillation performed by people with minimal training using automated external defibrillators and so the UK Department of Health has a 'defibrillators in public places' initiative in common with many other developed countries [20].

Outcome following in-hospital cardiac arrest depends very much on the condition of the patient. The more impaired organ systems there are, the less likely the patient is to survive. Non-shockable rhythms are more likely and these have a very poor prognosis. Fig. 8.8 illustrates this in graphical form, using data from a large UK audit of in-hospital cardiac arrests [21].

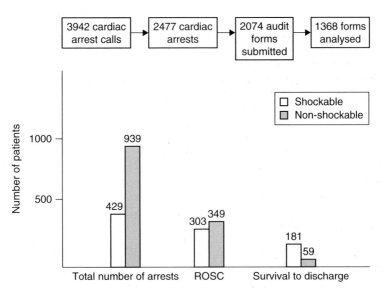

Figure 8.8 Outcome following in-hospital cardiac arrest. Data from 49 UK hospitals over a 6-month period. Of the cardiac arrests analysed, shockable rhythms (VF/VT) occurred in one-third and 181 out of 429 (40%) patients survived to discharge. For non-shockable rhythms (asystole/PEA), only 59 out of 939 (6%) patients survived to discharge. This data may exaggerate survival to discharge because only half of the cardiac arrests were analysed. ROSC: return of spontaneous circulation; VF: ventricular fibrillation; VT: ventricular tachycardia; PEA: pulseless electrical activity.

The UK guidelines on decisions relating to CPR [22] start with the words, 'CPR can be attempted on any person whose cardiac or respiratory functions cease. Failure of these functions is part of dying and thus CPR can theoretically be attempted on every individual prior to death. But because for every person there comes a time when death is inevitable, it is essential to identify patients for whom cardiopulmonary arrest represents a terminal event in their illness and in whom CPR is inappropriate. It is also essential to identify those patients who do not want CPR to be attempted and who competently refuse it.'

Communication around this area can be difficult. The UK guidelines set out a legal and ethical framework for CPR decisions. The British Medical Association Ethics Department has also produced a patient leaflet on CPR [23].

Various investigators have attempted to predict outcome following cardiac arrest based on physiological observations. One study looked at predictors of death and neurological outcome in 130 witnessed out-of-hospital cardiac arrest survivors presenting to an emergency department [24]. The investigators used time to return of spontaneous circulation, systolic BP at the time of presentation and a simple neurological examination to score patients. A prolonged cardiac arrest, with low BP and little neurological response following return of spontaneous circulation indicated an extremely poor prognosis.

Key points: brain failure

- Cerebral blood flow is affected by $PaCO_2$, PaO_2 and MAP.
- Secondary brain injury is preventable.
- Interventions designed to protect the brain from secondary injury improve outcome.
- In the unconscious patient, a systematic ABCDE approach is required.
- Prognosis following cardiac arrest is poor, unless there is a shockable rhythm and rapid access to defibrillation.

Self-assessment: case histories

1 A 20-year-old man is admitted unresponsive from a suspected heroin overdose. He receives 400 μg of i.v. naloxone in the emergency department and is sent up to the ward with a GCS of 15. You find him unresponsive, lying supine and snoring loudly. He has an oxygen mask on and the pulse oximeter shows his oxygen saturations are 99%. His other vital signs are: BP 110/60 mmHg, pulse 70/min, respiratory rate 5/min, temperature 37°C. How do you assess and manage him?

2 A 40-year-old man is found collapsed in his room with an empty bottle of tablets nearby. No other history is available. On examination his airway is clear, breathing is normal, BP is 80/40 mmHg and pulse is 130/min. The ECG shows a sinus tachycardia with a broad QRS complex. On neurological

examination he is unresponsive with reduced muscle tone, has intermittent jerking movements, bilateral up-going plantars, dilated pupils and a divergent strabismus. What is your management? Does he need a CT scan?

3 A 25-year-old builder has been hit on the head by machinery and is brought in unresponsive to the emergency department. There is a haematoma to the left side of his head. Airway is clear, breathing is normal and he is cardiovascularly stable (BP 140/70 mmHg and pulse 90/min). His GCS is calculated as 7 out of 15. What is your management?

4 A 70-year-old man is brought in with a dense left hemiplegia. His BP is 200/100 mmHg and his pulse is 75/min, sinus rhythm. A colleague calls you to ask whether this BP should be treated acutely and whether the patient has 'malignant hypertension'. What is your management?

5 A 30-year-old woman describes a sudden severe headache followed by vomiting. She has become drowsy on the way to hospital. You assess her GCS as 12. Outline your management priorities.

6 A 19-year-old man is brought in by ambulance having been found unresponsive by his girlfriend that morning. He went to bed the evening before complaining of flu-like symptoms and a headache. On examination he has a GCS of 8, respiratory rate 30/min, pulse 130/min, BP 70/40 mmHg and SpO_2 of 100% on 10 l/min oxygen via reservoir bag mask. There is neck stiffness and a faint purpuric rash on his trunk. What is your management?

7 A 70-year-old woman is brought into the emergency department having fallen off a step-ladder and injured her head. She has been lying on the floor for 12 h. Her vital signs on admission are: GCS 4, respiratory rate 10/min, pulse 30/min, BP 60/30 mmHg and temperature 29°C. Her arterial blood gases show: pH 7.2, $PaCO_2$ 6.0 kPa (46 mmHg), PaO_2 11.0 kPa (84.6 mmHg), st bicarbonate 17.2 mmol/l, base excess (BE) −12. What is your management? Why does she have these abnormal vital signs?

8 A 20-year-old man is admitted with increased frequency of seizures. He has had difficult to control epilepsy since childhood. So far he has had several brief partial seizures (episodes of staring). Following one of these he becomes unresponsive and his GCS is recorded as 5. What is the diagnosis and what is your management?

9 A 62-year-old post-operative man is resuscitated from a cardiac arrest, during which he required CPR for 20 min. Twenty-four hours after his cardiac arrest he has a heart rate of 100/min, BP 118/75 mmHg and a good urine output. Neurological examination reveals no pupillary reflexes, no spontaneous or roving eye movements and absent motor responses. What do you think about the neurological prognosis for this patient?

Self-assessment: discussion

1 This case illustrates that SpO_2 measurements are not a substitute for clinical assessment of airway and breathing. This patient has a partially obstructed airway and respiratory depression. Arterial blood gas analysis would reveal

a respiratory acidosis. All unconscious patients who are not intubated (e.g. post-ictal patients) should be nursed in the recovery position, attached to monitors and receive frequent clinical assessments. Naloxone i.v. has a short half-life. Repeated doses or an infusion may be used in this case.

2 In the first instance, manage ABC – fluid challenge(s). In D, check a capillary glucose and assess pupils for equal size and reactivity. In E, ask the paramedics what the empty bottle of tablets contained. These vital signs and neurological examination are characteristic of tricyclic poisoning. Sinus tachycardia with a broad QRS complex and hypotension is common in serious tricyclic poisoning and can sometimes be difficult to distinguish from ventricular tachycardia on a rhythm strip. Tricyclic poisoning accounts for half of the admissions to ICU with poisoning in the UK and it is a leading cause of death from drug overdose. Patients with a QRS width on the ECG of more than 160 ms are most at risk of cardiac arrhythmias and convulsions. The development of arrhythmias is potentiated by tachycardia, hypoxaemia and acidosis. Bradyarrythmias can also occur. Sodium bicarbonate i.v. acts as an antidote. Current recommendations are that 50–100 ml boluses of 8.4% sodium bicarbonate are given when the QRS duration is greater than 120 ms if there are serious arrhythmias or persistent hypotension (after securing the airway, giving oxygen and i.v. fluid) [25]. A CT scan of the brain is not indicated when there is a clear history and signs consistent with poisoning.

3 This patient should be managed by a team experience in Advanced Trauma and Life Support (ATLS). Management of A (airway) includes cervical spine control in this case. Tracheal intubation is indicated and the team will pay attention to preventing secondary brain injury using the measures outlined in Fig. 8.5. Once this patient is stable, he will be taken to CT scan and then either to a neuro-ICU or to a neurosurgical theatre.

4 Hypertension following stroke is a common response to brain ischaemia. Current practice is not to lower BP because blood supply to the potentially viable ischaemic penumbra could be compromised. In addition, many stroke patients are normally hypertensive so a 'normal' BP may in fact be too low. In this patient, attention must be paid to the airway, oxygen saturations, hydration, treatment of fever, lowering high glucose levels and nursing care. However, there are certain situations in which an *expert* would lower excessively high BP following a stroke caused by primary intracerebral haemorrhage, so seek advice. 'Malignant hypertension' is rare and the term 'hypertensive crisis' is better. Hypertensive crisis occurs either on a background of hypertensive disease or as part of other conditions: eclampsia, phaeochromocytoma and post-operatively (cardiac surgery). There is progressive severe hypertension with encephalopathy (confusion, headache, visual disturbances, fitting, reduced conscious level) and other end-organ damage: renal impairment and heart failure. If this occurs on a background of hypertensive disease, oral therapy is preferred as sudden dramatic falls in BP may cause organ damage through hypoperfusion.

5 This history is consistent with SAH. Management priorities here are A (ensure a patent airway and give oxygen), B (breathing) and C (circulation). For D, (disability), check pupil size and reactivity, a capillary glucose and GCS. A full neurological examination should be performed. Arterial blood gas analysis is helpful in assessing oxygenation, ventilation and perfusion, all important in the prevention of secondary brain injury. The patient should be transferred for an urgent CT brain scan. Patients with neurological signs (e.g. drowsiness) are likely to have an abnormal scan. When the diagnosis is confirmed, urgent transfer to a neurosurgical unit is required. The World Federation of Neurological Surgeons (WFNS) has devised a scale to compare the severity of SAH and this is shown in Fig. 8.9.

6 It is tempting to start with this case by being preoccupied with the diagnosis. But immediate management priorities are A (airway – call the anaesthetist), B (breathing) and C (circulation – give fluid challenges). In D, check pupils and capillary glucose. In E, give 2 g i.v. cefotaxime for meningococcal meningitis, and call for senior assistance if you have not done so already. The definitive management plan here includes tracheal intubation and ventilation, brain protection measures, an urgent CT brain scan, i.v. dexamethasone and samples for microbiology (but not LP). Close contacts require antibiotic prophylaxis. The UK guidelines on the management of meningococcal meningitis [26] are summarised in Fig. 8.10.

7 Management always start with A (airway – call the anaesthetist), B (breathing) and C (circulation – give fluid challenges and try atropine). But in this case, bear in mind the possibility of a cervical spine injury as elderly ladies are likely to have osteoporosis and she has fallen and sustained a head injury. In D (disability), check pupils for equal size and reactivity and check capillary glucose. In E, perform a thorough examination and gather what other history is available. In this case further investigations include urgent imaging of the head and neck, CK (creatine kinase), amylase and thyroid function (severe hypothyroidism can present with the same signs). Her abnormal vital signs are as a result of hypothermia, or spinal shock (a syndrome following sudden spinal cord injury characterised by hypotension and bradycardia if the cervical spine is affected). The patient should be warmed slowly and transferred to the ICU.

WFNS grade	GCS	Major focal neurological deficit
1	15	Absent
2	13–14	Absent
3	13–14	Present
4	7–12	Present or absent
5	3–6	Present or absent

Figure 8.9 World Federation of Neurological Surgeons SAH grading.

Meningococcal meningitis

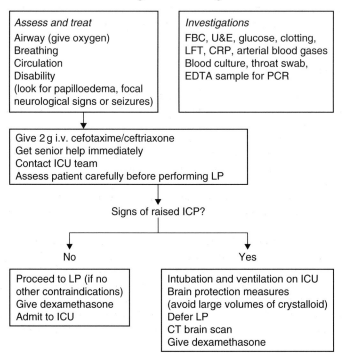

Figure 8.10 Summary of the management of meningococcal meningitis. Signs of raised ICP include confusion or altered conscious level, focal neurology, seizures, papilloedema, bradycardia and hypertension. A normal CT scan does not exclude raised ICP. Dexamethasone dose is 0.15 mg/kg qds for 4 days in adult bacterial meningitis. PCR: polymerise chain reaction.

8 The management still starts with ABC. D starts with pupil size and reactivity and capillary glucose measurement. A full examination and review of the history comes next. In this case, the likely diagnosis is non-convulsive status epilepticus, a condition which is under-recognised rather than rare [27]. Non-convulsive status is not associated with the same physiological disturbances (e.g. hypoxaemia, metabolic acidosis) as tonic–clonic status. Drug treatment is the same as for tonic–clonic status.

9 This patient has suffered global cerebral ischaemia during cardiac arrest. The best neurological recovery is seen in patients who have a short duration of coma. Patients who remain in a coma 7–14 days after global ischaemia are unlikely to ever become independent. Signs suggesting neurological recovery are related to certain brainstem reflexes on initial examination. Absent pupillary light reflexes (allowing for the effects of cardiac arrest drugs to have abated) place the patient in a very poor prognostic category. The presence of pupillary light reflexes with the return of spontaneous eye opening and conjugate eye movements accompanied by motor responses improves the prognosis and chance of independence. Based on this patient's examination at 24 h, independent function is very unlikely.

References

1. Marik P, Chen K, Varon J, Fromm Jr R and Sternbach GL. Management of increased intracranial pressure: a review for clinicians. *The Journal of Emergency Medicine* 1999; **17(4)**: 711–719.
2. Eker C, Asgeirsson B, Grande P-O, Schalen W and Nordstrom C-H. Improved outcome after severe head injury with a new therapy based on principles for brain volume regulation and preserved microcirculation. *Critical Care Medicine* 1998; **11**: 1881–1886.
3. Grande PO. Pathophysiology of brain insult. Therapeutic implications of the Lund Concept [Congress report]. *Schweizerische Medizinische Wochenschrift* 2000; **130**: 1538–1543.
4. McIntyre LA, Fergusson DA, Hebert PC, Moher D and Hutchinson JS. Prolonged therapeutic hypothermia after traumatic brain injury in adults: a systematic review. *Journal of American Medical Association* 2003; **289(22)**: 2992–2999.
5. Miller JD and Becker DP. Secondary insults to the injured brain. *Journal of the Royal College of Surgeons of Edinburgh* 1982; **27**: 292–298.
6. Jackson R and Butler J. Hypertonic or isotonic saline in hypotensive patients with severe head injury [Best evidence topic report]. *Emergency Medicine Journal* 2004; **21**: 80–81.
7. Bates D. Medical coma. In: Hughes RAC, ed. *Neurological Emergencies*, 4th edn. BMJ Books, London, 2003.
8. Scholtes FB, Renier WO and Meinhardi H. Non-convulsive status epilepticus: causes, treatment and outcome in 65 patients. *Journal of Neurology Neurosurgery and Psychiatry* 1996; **61**: 93–95.
9. Morgenstern LB, Luna-Gonzales H, Huber Jr JC *et al.* Worst headache and subarachnoid haemorrhage: prospective, modern computed tomography and spinal fluid analysis. *Annals of Emergency Medicine* 1998; **32**: 297–304.
10. Neil-Dwyer D and Lang D. 'Brain attack' – aneurysmal subarachnoid haemorrhage: death due to delayed diagnosis. *Journal of the Royal College of Physicians of London* 1997; **31**: 49–52.
11. www.i-h-s.org. International Headache Society website.
12. Edlow JA and Caplan L. Avoiding pitfalls in the diagnosis of subarachnoid haemorrhage [Review article]. *New England Journal of Medicine* 2000; **342(1)**: 29–36.
13. Vermeulen M. Subarachnoid haemorrhage. Diagnosis and treatment. *Journal of Neurology* 1996; **243**: 496–501.
14. Byrne JV, Molyneux AJ, Brennan RP *et al.* Embolisation of recently ruptured intracranial aneurysms. *Journal of Neurology Neurosurgery and Psychiatry* 1995; **59**: 616–620.
15. Mullner M. You should know, you're a medic: sudden cardiac death. *Student British Medical Journal* March 1999.
16. Diem SJ, Lantos JD and Tulsky JA. Cardiopulmonary resuscitation on television. Miracles and misinformation. *New England Journal of Medicine* 1996; **334**: 1578–1582.

17. Becker LB, Ostrander MP, Barrett J and Kondos GT. Outcome of cardiopulmonary resuscitation in a large metropolitan area: where are the survivors? *Annals of Emergency Medicine* 1991; **20**: 355–361.

18. Taffet GE, Teasdale TA and Luchi RJ. In-hospital cardiopulmonary resuscitation. *Journal of American Medical Association* 1988; **260**: 2069–2072.

19. Kimman GP, Ivens EM, Hartman JA, Hart HN and Simmons ML. Long term survival after successful out-of-hospital resuscitation. *Resuscitation* 1994; **28**: 227–232.

20. Davies CS, Colquhoun M, Graham S, Evans T and Chamberlain D. Defibrillators in public places: the introduction of a national scheme for public access defibrillation in England. *Resuscitation* 2002; **52**: 13–21.

21. Gwinnutt CL, Columb M and Harris R. Outcome after cardiac arrest in adults in UK hospitals: effect of the 1997 guidelines. *Resuscitation* 2000; **47**: 125–135.

22. www.bma.org.uk/ap.nsf/Content/cardioresus

23. www.bma.org.uk/ap.nsf/Content/Hubethics

24. Thompson RJ, McCullough PA, Kahn JK and O'Neill WW. Prediction of death and neurologic outcome in the emergency department in out-of-hospital cardiac arrest survivors. *American Journal of Cardiology* 1998; **81**: 17–21.

25. www.spib.axl.co.uk. Toxbase is the UK National Poisons Information Service website and is available in every UK accident and emergency department.

26. www.meningitis.org. The Meningitis Research Foundation UK website which contains useful information for health professionals including an algorithm and junior doctors' handbook.

27. Dunne JW, Summers QA and Stewart-Wynne EG. Non-convulsive status epilepticus: a prospective study in an adult general hospital. *Quarterly Journal of Medicine* 1987; **62(238)**: 117–126.

CHAPTER 9

Optimising patients before surgery

> **By the end of this chapter you will be able to:**
> - Understand peri-operative risk assessment
> - Understand the purpose of the medical consultation
> - Assess peri-operative risk in patients with cardiac disease
> - Assess peri-operative risk in patients with respiratory and other diseases
> - Understand the principles behind pre-operative optimisation
> - Apply this to your clinical practice

Risk assessment in the pre-operative patient

What is risk? In 1992, the Royal Society defined risk as 'the probability that a particular event occurs during a stated period of time, or results from a particular challenge' [1]. It defined a hazard as 'a situation that could lead to harm'.

How is surgical risk calculated? Many examples of risk prediction systems have been developed to enable surgical teams to assess and modify risk and allow informed consent for patients. These systems are designed to predict mortality and post-operative complications based on relevant prognostic factors including age, disease severity and co-morbidity.

Surgical practice also takes place within the context of clinical governance (a means by which the whole organisation ensures quality of care). In the UK, the establishment of the Commission for Health Improvement (CHI), National Institute for Clinical Excellence (NICE) and the National Clinical Assessment Authority (NCAA) has made it even more important for surgical teams to show that they are following evidence-based practices that offer the best standard of care to their patients.

The National Confidential Enquiry into Patient Outcome and Death (NCEPOD), now part of the National Patient Safety Agency (NPSA), produces regular national audits which have studied deaths within the first 30 days after surgery. The report in 2003 reaffirmed the view that patients do better and risks are minimised when:
- They are operated on by specialists with high-volume experience in that field of surgery.

- They are cared for in environments where all essential services are provided on one site.
- They are cared for in environments where all emergency patients have prompt access to theatres, critical care facilities and appropriately trained staff 24 h a day every day of the year.

Of the 3 million operations performed in the UK each year, NCEPOD reported that there were over 20,000 deaths following surgery.

Examples of risk prediction systems

The following are commonly used to predict peri-operative risk:
- American Society of Anaesthesiologists (ASA) classification of disease severity
- Acute physiological and chronic health evaluation (APACHE) score
- Simplified acute physiological score (SAPS)
- Physiological and operative severity score for the enumeration of mortality and morbidity (POSSUM).

The ASA classification divides patients into five categories according to their general medical history and examination without the need for any specific tests. Although it is not a sensitive predictor of mortality, there is general correlation with overall outcome following surgery, and it is used in clinical trials to standardise disease severity. Fig. 9.1 outlines the ASA classification, which is also used to predict outcome in specific conditions (e.g. colon cancer).

The APACHE score is now in its third form and involves scoring several acute physiological variables added to a score derived from age and any chronic health problems. It is used worldwide in ICUs to score the severity of illness on admission and is also used for audit. The APACHE score has been extensively validated and is a reliable method of estimating ICU mortality for

Class	Characteristics	General peri-operative mortality (%)	Mortality in large bowel obstruction due to cancer (%)
1	Healthy patient	0.05	2.6
2	Mild systemic disease which does not limit function	0.4	7.6
3	Moderate systematic disease which limits function	4.5	23.9
4	Severe systemic disease which is a constant threat to life	25	42
5	Moribund patient who will not survive 24 h without surgery	50	66.7

Figure 9.1 ASA classification of disease severity. Extremes of age, smoking and pregnancy are criteria for ASA 2. The addition of the postscript E denotes emergency surgery.

groups of patients. Its use in elective surgical patients is of uncertain value. The acute physiological variables include: vital signs, arterial pH and key blood results (sodium, potassium, creatinine, haematocrit and white cell count). The more abnormal these are, the more points are given. Points are added for age and chronic ill health, for example liver disease, heart failure, chronic lung disease, dialysis or immunocompromised. As with all scoring systems, the APACHE score has to be used in context. For example, some patients with high scores on admission have low mortality rates, for example diabetic ketoacidosis, and some patients with low scores on admission have high mortality rates, for example intracranial haemorrhage. Fig. 9.2 shows the probability of death in hospital based on APACHE score on admission to ICU [2,3].

The SAPS score is a derivation of the APACHE score and is assigned 24 h after admission. It uses a mathematical formula to give a numerical value of the predicted hospital mortality rate.

The POSSUM scoring system is used by many surgeons in the UK [4,5]. It is more detailed than the ASA classification but less complicated than the APACHE score. It has been developed for different types of surgery and uses 12 physiological variables and 6 operative variables to derive a score. Originally it was used as a tool to compare morbidity and mortality between different surgical techniques. It is now used to estimate post-operative morbidity and mortality. The physiological variables in POSSUM include: age, heart rate, BP, Glasgow Coma Score, the presence of cardiac signs, abnormalities on the ECG, any respiratory problems and key blood test results. The operative variables include urgency, malignancy, peritoneal soiling, blood loss, re-operation and severity of surgery.

Communicating risk

Despite scoring systems, it is often very difficult to communicate risk to individual patients in a meaningful way. Individuals tend to evaluate risk based on many subjective aspects rather than statistical data. The assessment and perception of risk is subconscious, subjective, personality dependent and fails to follow any rational or methodical pattern.

APACHE score	Mortality (%)
0–5	2.3
6–10	4.3
11–15	8.6
16–20	16.4
21–25	28.6
26–30	56.4
31+	70

Figure 9.2 Hospital mortality based on APACHE score on admission to ICU.

Patients are frequently anxious or frightened before surgery, especially emergency surgery. Many doctors are afraid they will exacerbate this by discussing risk. However, studies have shown that anxiety levels are not increased when information about the risks of anaesthesia and surgery and its complications are discussed in detail with patients prior to any surgical intervention. Recent medico-legal cases have also emphasised that all patients should receive sufficient information, in a way that they can understand, in order to enable them to make informed decisions about their care. Therefore, it is important that risks are discussed before surgery and not withheld for fear of upsetting the patient [6].

What does a 1:1000 risk of death mean to an individual patient? Some risk scales have been devised that are more easily understood by patients, by comparing the risks of surgery and anaesthesia to risks associated with some activities of daily living that people readily accept [7]. One example is shown in Fig. 9.3.

Once the risks of surgery have been assessed, the risks vs benefits need to be considered. If the risks outweigh the benefits, surgery may have to be reconsidered. If surgery is necessary, the patient should be told about serious and commonly occurring risks. The most common surgical diagnoses in patients who die after an operation are: fractured neck of femur, colorectal cancer, occlusive peripheral vascular disease, aortic aneurysm, mesenteric ischaemia, peptic ulceration and diverticulitis.

The medical consultation

Physiological reserve is an important concept in patients facing major or emergency surgery and in critical illness. The cardiovascular system in particular has to mount a compensatory response to the physiological stress which occurs. Patients who lack the ability to mount a response have increased mortality.

Physicians are asked to assess many patients prior to surgery. The specific reason for this is to help in the assessment of peri-operative risk and to optimise the patient's medical condition. It is not the role of the physician to say whether a patient is fit for anaesthesia, that is the role of the anaesthetist. If the patient's condition is optimised as much as possible, he will be more able to deal with the physiological stress of surgery.

The key components of the medical consultation are:
- To find out the severity of the disease in question
- Understand the type of surgery and anaesthesia being proposed
- Specifically recommend measures to treat the disease, optimise the patient's condition and reduce peri-operative risk
- Plan post-operative care with colleagues.

If you are asking a physician for a pre-operative visit, it is important that you think of these components and request clearly what it is you want him to address, for example can this patient's condition be improved?

Risk level	Verbal description	UK community examples of risk	Anaesthetic/surgical examples of risk
1:1 ↓	Very common	Death from a heart attack	Post-operative nausea and vomiting 1:4 Dizziness 1:5 Headache 1:5
1:10 ↓	Common	Winning three balls in the national lottery	Oral trauma following tracheal intubation 1:20 Emergency surgery death 1:40 Difficult intubation 1:50
1:100 ↓	Uncommon	Death from smoking	Peri-operative death 1:200 Failure to intubate 1:500 Awareness without pain in anaesthesia 1:300
1:1000 ↓	Rare	Death from road traffic accident	Awareness with pain in anaesthesia 1:3000 Aspiration 1:3000 Cardiac arrest (regional anaesthesia) 1:3000 Epidural abscess 1:5000 Failure to intubate and ventilate 1:5000
1:10,000 ↓	Very rare	Death by murder	Anaphylaxis 1:10,000 Cardiac arrest (general anaesthesia) 1:15,000 Death related to anaesthesia 1:50,000
1:100,000 ↓	Extremely rare	Death by rail accident	Loss of vision (general anesthesia) 1:125,000 Paraplegia (regional anaesthesia) 1:100,000 Epidural haematoma 1:150,000 Death solely due to anaesthesia 1:200,000
1:1 million ↓	Negligible	Winning the national lottery	HIV infection from blood transfusion
1:10 million		Death from being struck by lightning	

Figure 9.3 Scales of risk.

The assessment of patients with cardiac disease

The largest single cause of peri-operative death is cardiac related, therefore much research has been done to try to assess cardiovascular risk before surgery.

The main types of cardiac disease that patients present with before surgery are:
- Ischaemic heart disease
- Heart failure

Minor (Risk factors for coronary artery disease)	Intermediate (Stable coronary artery disease)	Major (Unstable coronary artery disease)
• Family history of ischaemic heart disease • Uncontrolled hypertension • High-cholestrol • Smoker • Abnormal ECG • Previous myocardial infarction or CABG, asymptomatic on no treatment	• Myocardial infarction or CABG within 3 months • Angina (NYHA class 1–2) • Documented previous perioperative cardiac ischaemia • Previous myocardial infarction, asymptomatic on treatment • Diabetes • Age >70 • Compensated or previous heart failure	• Myocardial infarction or CABG within 6 weeks • Angina (NYHA class 3–4) • Decompensated heart failure • Significant arrhythmias

Figure 9.4 Patient risk factors which predict peri-operative cardiac complications.

- Valve disease
- Atrial fibrillation (AF)
- Hypertension
- Patients with pacemakers.

Ischaemic heart disease

The overall incidence of peri-operative cardiac events is <10%. But, certain patients have a higher risk and targeted testing and modification of risk factors improves outcome in this group. Despite a number of tests available which can help to assess risk, the key to evaluating a patient's risk of peri-operative cardiac ischaemia is a careful history, examination and 12-lead ECG.

Peri-operative myocardial infarction is caused either by a rupture of coronary atherosclerotic plaque and thrombus formation (similar to a non-operative setting) or a mismatch between myocardial oxygen supply and demand. Factors that increase myocardial oxygen demand are mainly as a result of peri-operative stress: tachycardia, hypertension, pain, interruption of usual cardiac medication or the use of sympathomimetic drugs. Factors which reduce myocardial oxygen supply include hypotension, anaemia and hypoxaemia.

There are three components to assessing patients with coronary artery disease before non-cardiac surgery:

1 Patient risk factors
2 Surgical risk factors
3 Functional capacity of the patient.

Fig. 9.4 shows the minor, intermediate and major patient risk factors which predict peri-operative cardiac complications. Fig. 9.5 shows the risk associated with different procedures.

Low risk	Intermediate risk	High risk
• Endoscopic procedures • Day case surgery • Superficial procedures • Eye surgery • Plastic surgery • Breast surgery	• Carotid endarterectomy • ENT • Neurosurgery • Abdominal • Thoracic • Orthopaedic • Prostate	• Emergency major surgery • Aortic and major vascular surgery • Prolonged procedure with large fluid shifts or blood loss

Figure 9.5 Risk associated with different procedures.

One of the most useful measures with regard to ischaemic heart disease is the patient's functional capacity [8]. Risk is increased in patients who cannot reach four metabolic equivalents (METs) of workload. One MET is equivalent to the oxygen consumption of a resting 40-year-old 70 kg man. Climbing a flight of stairs, walking up a hill, briskly walking on the flat, mowing the lawn, swimming or playing a round of golf is at least four METs. The inability to climb two flights of stairs is associated with a positive predictive value of 90% for post-operative cardiopulmonary complications, such as myocardial infarction, after high-risk surgery [9].

The American College of Cardiology and American Heart Association has produced evidence-based guidelines on peri-operative cardiovascular evaluation for non-cardiac surgery [10]. A much more simplified algorithm is shown in Fig. 9.6. To summarise, low-risk patients with good functional capacity who are undergoing low-or intermediate-risk surgery can proceed without further evaluation. Intermediate risk patients require evaluation if they have poor functional capacity, or are undergoing major surgery. All high-risk patients require further evaluation.

Other cardiac risk assessments include the Lee Score [11], derived from the prospective observation of nearly 3000 patients and used six independent predictors of cardiac risk. Fig. 9.7 shows the relationship between the number of risk factors and the likelihood of peri-operative adverse cardiac events.

The Goldman cardiac risk index [12] is another well known indicator of cardiac risk, based on observational data from 1000 patients and the Detsky score [13] is a later modification of this. These use variables based on history, examination, blood results and the 12-lead ECG.

Further evaluation in high-risk patients is required to assess the degree of and treatment options for their disease, if this will change the management of the case. The surgical management can be modified by changing:

• Drug therapy
• The planned surgical treatment

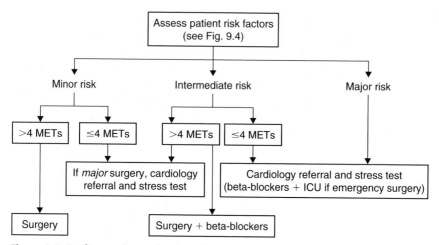

Figure 9.6 Cardiovascular evaluation of patients prior to non-cardiac surgery.

Number of risk factors	Population (%)	Adverse cardiac events (%)
0	36	0.4
1	39	0.9
2	18	7
3 or more	7	11

Figure 9.7 The Lee Score. Risk factors: high-risk surgery; ischaemic heart disease; heart failure; cerebrovascular disaease; diabetes; creatinine above 175 μmol/l (2.1 mg/dl).

- The anaesthetic technique
- The patient's understanding of risks vs benefits and wishes.

Further evaluation involves referral to a cardiologist and investigations, such as stress testing. Often non-exercise tests are performed as many high-risk surgical patients cannot exercise sufficiently. Dobutamine stress testing is one example, which has a negative predictive value of almost 100%, although a low-positive predictive value in terms of peri-operative risk [8]. Depending on the results of stress testing, patients may benefit from coronary revascularisation, or simply modification of their peri-operative care.

It used to be the rule to wait 6 months after a myocardial infarction before non-cardiac surgery. However, risk after a previous myocardial infarction is related more to the functional status of the patient and the amount of myocardium at risk from further ischaemia rather than the age of the infarction. In uncomplicated cases, there is no benefit in delaying surgery by more than 3 months.

Vascular surgery poses particular cardiac risks because many of the risk factors for peripheral vascular disease are the same for coronary artery disease (diabetes, smoking and hyperlipidaemia). Asymptomatic coronary artery disease is common in vascular patients and cardiac symptoms may be masked by the limited mobility of these patients. The diagnosis of myocardial infarction in the peri-operative period can be difficult as half of patients do not have typical chest pain. They may present with arrhythmias, pulmonary oedema, hypotension or confusion. ECG changes, usually T-wave abnormalities, are common post-operatively and do not necessarily indicate myocardial infarction. Troponin measurement is helpful in these circumstances.

Beta-blockers in the peri-operative period

The peri-operative period is associated with prolonged sympathetic stimulation which increases myocardial oxygen demand. Several randomised trials have looked at medical therapy (e.g. nitrates, beta-blockers) to reduce peri-operative cardiovascular risk. The intra-operative use of nitroglycerin in high-risk patients does not affect outcome despite reduced ischaemia on the ECG. Some trials have showed that peri-operative beta-blockers reduce cardiac complications and mortality. In a study with vascular patients, cardiac mortality and morbidity was reduced by bisoprolol from 34% to 3.4% [14]. As a consequence of such trials, beta-blockers have been recommended for high-risk patients and patients with hypertension, ischaemic heart disease or risk factors for ischaemic heart disease. It has also been recommended that if pre-operative administration is not possible, an i.v. beta-blocker given at induction of anaesthesia followed by post-operative treatment should be used.

However, a recent meta-analysis has concluded that the evidence on peri-operative beta-blockers is encouraging but too unreliable to allow definitive conclusions to be drawn [15]. Twenty two clinical trials involving 2437 patients were analysed. Several different beta-blockers were used in several different ways. More conclusive evidence is awaited from the POISE (peri-operative ischaemic evaluation) trial [16].

Heart failure

The ejection fraction, as measured by echocardiography, is one measure of cardiac functional reserve. A reduced ejection fraction also correlates with an increased risk of peri-operative pulmonary oedema.

It has long been observed that high-risk patients who survive surgery have greater compensatory increases in cardiac output and oxygen delivery than patients who die. Non-survivors are unable to compensate for the added metabolic and cardiorespiratory demands of surgery. This has led to the concept of pre-operative optimisation whereby pre-operative interventions to improve cardiac function and oxygen delivery are used. Pre-operative optimisation is discussed further in a Mini-tutorial.

Valve disease

Severe aortic stenosis (AS) is the most difficult valve problem in the peri-operative period. AS is a fixed obstruction and limits maximum cardiac output during stress. Patients cannot respond normally to the peripheral dilatation associated with anaesthesia and BP can fall dramatically. This causes myocardial ischaemia as the myocardial hypertrophy seen in AS is associated with increased oxygen demand. AS may be asymptomatic and elderly patients with severe stenosis may not necessarily exhibit classical features on examination.

Mitral stenosis is also important to recognise because it is necessary to control the heart rate in order to preserve diastole in this condition. The left atrium fills in diastole, generating enough pressure to squeeze blood through the stenosed valve. The presence of any murmur requires a pre-operative echocardiogram. Antibiotic prophylaxis may also be required.

Atrial fibrillation

Arrhythmias following surgery are common, often exacerbated by the abrupt withdrawal of cardiac drugs due to fasting. They are also caused by hypotension, metabolic acidosis and hypoxaemia, all of which can be prevented. It is important that patients with heart disease are maintained on their usual drugs, via alternative routes if feasible, during the peri-operative period.

Five per cent patients over the age of 65 have chronic AF and it is a common pre-operative finding. Certain procedures are also associated with the development of AF, for example intrathoracic surgery. Patients with chronic lung or cardiac disease are at greater risk of developing post-operative AF. The main difference in the pre-operative period is that beta- or calcium-channel blockers and amiodarone are more effective than digoxin in controlling the ventricular rate during stress. If the patient is anti-coagulated, this also needs to be addressed in the pre-operative period.

Hypertension

The risks of pre-operative hypertension are unclear, with some studies showing increased cardiovascular complications and others no increased risk. Hypertension alone is therefore considered a borderline risk factor. Uncontrolled or poorly controlled hypertension can be associated with increased intra-operative complications, such as myocardial ischaemia, arrhythmias, stroke and exaggerated swings in BP. There is no clear evidence that deferring surgery in such patients reduces peri-operative risk, but many anaesthetists would postpone elective surgery in a hypertensive patient because the potential risks may outweigh the benefits.

Patients with pacemakers

Patients with pacemakers are commonly encountered in theatre and generally do not pose a problem. ECG and chest X-ray should be requested to confirm the type and integrity of the pacemaker. It should also be checked by the cardiology team prior to surgery to ensure that it is functioning correctly. Patients with a high degree of heart block on pre-operative ECG (bi or trifascicular block) should be considered for prophylactic temporary pacing prior to surgery.

Mini-tutorial: cardiopulmonary exercise testing

Many of the assessments used in the pre-operative evaluation of patients prior to surgery are based on variables, such as age and past medical history and give useful information about overall mortality and morbidity. However, this does not provide individualised information for a particular patient. Cardiopulmonary exercise (CPX) testing is an inexpensive, non-invasive pre-operative test which mimics the peri-operative increase in oxygen demand required for major surgery and correlates well with post-operative outcome.

It is easier to spot patients who are at risk of myocardial ischaemia, either on the basis of history, the resting 12-lead ECG or vascular-risk factors, but it has long been recognised that there is another group of patients at risk of adverse cardiac events, those whose hearts cannot meet the physiological demands of surgery. This is discussed further in the Mini-tutorial on Pre-optimisation of high-risk surgical patients.

In one study [17], all patients over the age of 60 years or those with a history of ischaemic heart disease or heart failure underwent CPX testing prior to major surgery. The results of the CPX test were then used to triage 620 patients for admission to ICU, high dependency unit (HDU) or the ward. All patients undergoing aortic or oesophageal surgery were automatically scheduled for ICU admission. On the basis of CPX testing, high-risk patients were admitted to ICU pre-operatively for optimisation and returned to ICU after surgery. 28% of patients were triaged to ICU, 21% to HDU and 51% to the ward. In-hospital cardiovascular mortality was 4.7% in the ICU group, 1.7% in the HDU group and 0% in the ward group, showing that CPX testing had a high-predictive value.

Following a resting 12-lead ECG and baseline respiratory function tests, the patient is asked to exercise on a bicycle ergometer while breathing in and out of a mouthpiece. Inspired and expired gases are sampled and analysed by computer for oxygen consumption and carbon dioxide (CO_2) production. The patient is asked to pedal against an increasing resistance. The anaerobic threshold (AT) occurs when the ability to meet energy requirements through aerobic metabolism is exceeded. It is detected when the rate of increase of CO_2 production exceeds the rate of increase of oxygen consumption. The higher the AT, the fitter the patient. AT is an accurate measure of cardiac function, is independent of the motivation of the patient and occurs well before the maximum aerobic capacity. It can be measured easily as it does not require high physical stress. An AT of <11 ml/kg/min is associated with an increase in peri-operative cardiovascular deaths.

CPX testing measures cardiorespiratory reserve as well as myocardial ischaemia. Although not yet in widespread clinical use in the UK, it is used commonly to evaluate the fitness of athletes and the condition of patients prior to cardiac transplantation.

The assessment of patients with respiratory and other diseases

Obstructive lung diseases are the most commonly encountered pulmonary problems in anaesthetic practice. At pre-operative assessment, the presence of dyspnoea or wheezing should alert the clinician that the patient's condition is not well controlled. Cessation of smoking prior to surgery should be encouraged as there are both immediate and long-term benefits, such as reduction in oxygen demand, reduced airway reactivity, increase in ciliary motility and a reduced risk of post-operative chest infections.

Pre-operative lung function tests and arterial blood gases can quantify the type and degree of respiratory impairment and predict the need for post-operative ventilatory support. High-risk patients include those who are breathless at rest, have a $PaCO_2$ greater than 6.0 kPa (46 mmHg), a forced expiratory volume (FEV_1) <1 l or an FEV_1/FVC (forced vital capacity) ratio of <50%.

Other factors which make pulmonary complications more likely include:
- High ASA class
- Chronic obstructive pulmonary disease (COPD)
- Smoking within the previous 8 weeks
- Surgery lasting longer than 3 h
- Obesity
- Upper abdominal or thoracic surgery.

Certain measures help to reduce peri-operative pulmonary complications. As well as smoking cessation, these are pre-operative inhaled beta-agonists for patients with COPD, or steroids if needed, the use of regional anaesthesia (with or without general anaesthesia) and post-operative lung expansion exercises.

Obesity

Morbid obesity is defined as over twice the ideal body weight, or a body mass index of more than 30 kg/m^2. Approximately 20% of adults in the UK are obese by this definition and this figure continues to rise. Obesity poses significant problems during anaesthesia and surgery. There are physiological differences in obese patients: increased oxygen demand and CO_2 production with increased ventilation as a result, reduced lung compliance, increased cardiac output and a greater incidence of hypertension, sleep apnoea and diabetes. Special equipment may be needed (e.g. theatre trolleys), venous access is difficult and non-invasive BP measurements are often inaccurate.

From an anaesthetic point of view, airway management and intubation of the trachea can be difficult and gastro-oesophageal reflux is usually present, increasing the risk of aspiration. Ventilation of obese patients can be difficult and they decompensate more quickly during apnoea. Drug doses based on ideal body weight can be difficult to calculate and the distribution and metabolism of anaesthetic drugs is altered. Regional anaesthetic techniques, for example epidural are difficult to perform. Surgery is also more likely to be technically difficult.

Obesity is associated with an increased risk of post-operative complications, such as venous thromboembolism and respiratory failure. Patients weighing more than 115 kg (250 lbs) are twice as likely to develop post-operative pneumonia. An awareness of the problems that obesity poses is important. The anaesthetist should be informed about obese patients, even if they have no other past medical history. These patients also require close monitoring during the post-operative period, with particular attention paid to thromboembolism prophylaxis, effective analgesia and early mobilisation.

Diabetes

Diabetes mellitus is a common condition, affecting just over 1% of the western European population. Still more people have undiagnosed type 2 diabetes. The high incidence of this disease, together with many of the complications of the disease requiring surgical intervention, means that many diabetic patients will present for surgery and some will need detailed assessment and management.

Diabetic patients have a higher post-operative risk for the following:
- Nausea and vomiting
- Aspiration because of gastroparesis
- Pulmonary complications
- Disrupted diabetic control
- Heel pressure sores due to peripheral neuropathy
- Wound infection
- Myocardial infarction
- Cardiac arrest
- Acute renal failure
- Stroke.

Therefore, the pre-operative history should include details about the type and treatment of diabetes, known complications (especially ischaemic heart disease, renal impairment or peripheral vascular disease) and previous hospital admissions. Examination should look specifically for evidence of heart disease or hypertension. The presence of orthostatic hypotension may indicate autonomic neuropathy and the potential for cardiac complications. Abnormal creatinine and urinalysis may indicate diabetic nephropathy. Haemoglobin A_{1C} (HbA_{1C}) measurements indicate whether or not blood sugar has been well controlled.

Specific instructions on the peri-operative control of blood glucose vary between specialists and institutions. Insulin is an anabolic hormone that is opposed by the catabolic effects of catecholamines, cortisol, glucagon and growth hormone. In the fasting state insulin secretion decreases and catabolic hormones levels rise leading to hyperglycaemia and ketoacidosis. Similarly, surgery elicits a stress response that is directly related to the degree of trauma. Levels of catecholamines and cortisol rise producing insulin hyposecretion, insulin resistance and increased protein catabolism. Providing a baseline glucose infusion together with insulin replacement reduces protein catabolism and restores glucose and electrolyte balance. The aim in peri-operative

10% glucose + 10 mmol KCl at 50 ml/h

plus 50 units soluble insulin (Actrapid) in 50 ml 0.9% saline as prescribed below:

Insulin sliding scale			
Blood sugar (mmol/l)	Units insulin/h Gentle regimen	Units insulin/h Standard regimen	Units insulin/h Aggressive regimen
<3.5 or signs of hypoglycaemia – give 25 ml i.v. 50% dextrose and call doctor			
<4.0	0.25	0.5	1
4.0–9	0.5	1	2
9.1–11	1	2	4
11.1–17	2	3	8
17.1–28	4	4	10
>28	6 and call doctor to review regimen	6 and call doctor to review regimen	12 and call doctor to review regimen/refer to diabetic team

- Monitor blood glucose hourly for 6 h then 2 h if stable
- Monitor electrolytes

Figure 9.8 An example i.v. insulin regime.

diabetic patients is to maintain a normal blood glucose (4–8 mmol/l). This is done by:
- Minimising fasting by placing patients first on the surgical list
- Monitoring glucose levels regularly
- Switching poorly controlled or acutely ill diabetics to an i.v. insulin regime
- Tailoring the diabetic plan to the type of anaesthetic and surgery.

In tablet controlled diabetes, patients should be switched to short acting drugs if possible. On the day of surgery their medication is omitted and glucose is monitored to ensure that it does not rise above 12 mmol/l. For major surgery or prolonged fasting, an i.v. insulin regime is recommended until the patient is eating and drinking normally.

In insulin dependent diabetes, patients have their usual insulin omitted on the day of surgery and are started on an i.v. insulin regime (this may not be necessary in minor surgery). After surgery, this is continued until the patient is eating and drinking normally. Fig. 9.8 shows an example regime.

Basic pre-operative optimisation

Rarely, surgery takes precedence over full resuscitation (e.g. in ruptured abdominal aortic aneurysm). In most cases there is time to resuscitate the patient. Pre-operative volume depletion is common and is exacerbated by regional or general anaesthetic drugs. Pre-operative volume losses occur due to:
- Vomiting
- Fasting

Mini-tutorial: pre-optimisation of high-risk surgical patients

Major surgery, especially emergency surgery, is a huge physiological stress on the body. As well as increasing oxygen demand, it generates a strong inflammatory response which increases oxygen requirements. Most patients can meet these demands by increasing cardiac output, but patients who are already compromised by cardio-respiratory disease, or the elderly, may not have this physiological reserve. This is the group of patients which faces the greatest risk of post-operative complications and death.

Bland and Shoemaker observed a mortality of 25% in their own high-risk surgical patients [18]. High-risk patients were those with poor pre-operative status about to undergo a major surgical procedure. Outcome was dramatically influenced by the ability of the patient's cardio-pulmonary system to adapt. Values for cardiac output, oxygen delivery and oxygen uptake were significantly higher in survivors than in non-survivors. It was postulated that the observed increase in cardiac output and oxygen delivery were physiological responses to increased peri-operative oxygen demand.

Based on this observation, one study randomised 88 patients into three groups: a standard group managed using a central venous pressure (CVP) line, a Pulmonary artery (PA) catheter group in which treatments were given to achieve normal values of cardiac output and oxygen delivery, and another PA catheter group in which treatments were given to achieve supranormal values of cardiac output and oxygen delivery [19]. Patients were treated prior to surgery using fluids or blood, inotropes and vasodilators, but in many cases fluids alone achieved the targets. The study demonstrated reduced mortality, complications and length of ICU stay in the supranormal group. Further studies ensued [20,21], which showed that pre-operative optimisation of cardiac output and oxygen delivery in high-risk surgical patients significantly improved outcome. There has been subsequent debate as to whether the goals should be normal or supranormal, as later studies showed adverse outcomes with supranormal targets.

The role of dopexamine

Boyd et al. [20] used dopexamine as their inotrope and Wilson et al. [21] compared dopexamine with adrenaline in pre-operative optimisation, with favourable results. Dopexamine (see Chapter 6) has anti-inflammatory properties and is a beta-2 agonist which causes an increase in heart rate and cardiac output as well as peripheral vasodilatation and an increase in renal and splanchnic blood flow. Cardiac output is increased as a result of afterload reduction and inotropy. In comparison to other inotropes, dopexamine causes the least increase in myocardial oxygen consumption.

Recently, the role of the gut in the pathogenesis of post-operative complications has been studied. Intramucosal pH (pH_i) has been used to monitor trauma patients instead of oxygen delivery via a PA catheter. Low gastric pH_i and increased gastric CO_2 levels predict post-operative complications [22]. This is thought to relate to gut hypoperfusion which causes bacterial translocation into the circulation, which precipitates a systemic inflammatory response syndrome and organ dysfunction. Dopexamine increases splanchnic blood flow and may have a protective role in this respect.

All of these and other studies support the simple concept that adequate fluid resuscitation is of vital importance in high-risk surgical patients.

- Bleeding
- Fluid loss into an obstructed bowel
- Sepsis or systemic inflammatory response syndrome (SIRS).

As stated throughout this book, optimal resuscitation makes a big difference to outcome. One should aim to restore the observations as far towards the patient's normal as possible before surgery. This is so that they can mount their best compensatory response during the peri-operative period.

Pre-operative aims should therefore be:

- Normal airway
- Normal respiratory rate
- PaO_2 more than 10 kPa (77 mmHg)
- Well perfused with good cardiac output
- Urine output more than 1 ml/kg/h
- Normal haemoglobin
- Normal glucose and electrolytes (especially K^+ and Mg^{2+})
- Normal base excess (BE).

As usual, these are simple airway, breathing and circulation (ABC) measures.

Key points: optimising patients before surgery

- There are many different examples of peri-operative risk prediction systems.
- The largest single cause of peri-operative death is cardiac related.
- Obesity and diabetes are also major problems.
- High-risk patients undergoing major surgery can be identified and pre-optimised in order to improve outcome.
- Basic resuscitation (ABC) prior to surgery is important.

Self-assessment: case histories

1 A 75-year-old woman has been admitted 24 h ago with large bowel obstruction. She is warm and tachycardic and had been unwell at home for several days before coming to hospital. Her urine output per hour has slowly reduced throughout the day and is now <0.5 ml/kg/h. Her other vital signs are: alert, pulse 100/min, BP 110/70 mmHg, respiratory rate 28/min, SpO_2 98% on 2 l nasal cannulae, temperature 37.5°C. She is listed for the acute theatre. What is your management?

2 A 70-year-old woman is due for a partial gastrectomy for stomach cancer but, the surgeons have noted that her ECG has changed compared with 4 weeks ago. There is new T-wave inversion in leads V1–V4. A physician is asked to decide whether or not she has had a myocardial infarction. She says she had an hour of chest discomfort 2 weeks ago, but did not seek medical attention. She does not suffer from angina or breathlessness, and is walking around the hospital with no symptoms. What is her peri-operative risk, what can be done to reduce that risk and what advice might the physician give?

3 A 60-year-old man comes to the pre-operative orthopaedic assessment clinic. He has a history of ischaemic heart disease and had a myocardial infarction many years ago. He does not have angina nowadays, on treatment. He arrives using a walking stick because of his painful knee, which is due to be replaced. Is it safe to proceed with the planned surgery in view of his heart disease? How do you assess this patient?

4 A 75-year-old woman is admitted following a fall and fractured left neck of femur. There is no past medical history. She has been lying on the floor for 18 h at home. On examination her skin feels warm and dry. She has the following vital signs: drowsy and in pain, pulse 110/min, BP 110/60 mmHg, respiratory rate 26/min, temperature 38°C, SpO$_2$ 92% on air, and has not passed urine since admission (not catheterised). There are coarse crackles at the left base of the lungs and a chest X-ray film shows pneumonia. She is listed for the trauma theatre as soon as possible. What do you need to do before she goes to theatre?

5 You are asked to see a 60-year-old man who is being booked for an elective inguinal hernia repair. In the out-patient clinic it is noted that his oxygen saturations are 89% on air and he is breathless on exertion. You are asked to advise on his chest condition before surgery. Further history reveals that he is a lifelong smoker and used to be a miner. He has been breathless on exertion for several years but has never seen a doctor. On examination he has hyper-expanded lungs and prolonged expiration with scattered wheeze. His chest X-ray film shows clear lung fields. His arterial blood gases on air show: pH 7.4, PaCO$_2$ 6.0 kPa (46 mmHg), PaO$_2$ 7.5 kPa (57.6 mmHg), st bicarbonate 27 mmol/l and BE +1. What is your advice?

6 A 65-year-old woman is admitted with small bowel obstruction, which is being treated conservatively with a nasogastric tube and i.v. fluids. She has a history of stable angina and hypertension. Her usual medication includes atenolol 50 mg a day. You are asked to see her urgently because her pulse is 140/min (previously 60/min). The ECG shows AF. Why has this happened and what is your management?

7 A 60-year-old man on treatment for angina and heart failure is admitted with bowel obstruction. He has been unwell with vomiting for 4 days. On examination he is alert with a pulse of 100/min, BP 100/50 mmHg, respiratory rate 24/min, SpO$_2$ 95% on air and temperature 37.5°C. His blood results show a raised white cell count, urea of 15 mmol/l (blood urea nitrogen (BUN) 41 mg/dl) and creatinine 300 μmol/l (3.6 mg/dl). His urea and creatinine were normal 3 months ago. He is listed for the acute theatre as soon as possible. What is your management?

Self-assessment: discussion

1 As always, management starts with A (airway and oxygen), B (breathing) and C (circulation). There are signs of hypoperfusion: increased respiratory rate, tachycardia, low BP and poor urine output. What is her normal BP?

The history, as well as examination, points towards volume depletion. Vomiting may have also caused hypokalaemia. She requires fluid resuscitation and close monitoring. Inform the anaesthetist, who may request more sophisticated monitoring to guide fluid and other therapies before surgery.

2 Myocardial infarction is diagnosed by history, ECG changes and a cardiac enzyme rise. Two out of three indicates a probable recent myocardial infarction. This, and the type of surgery, places the patient at high risk of peri-operative cardiac complications but, as the surgery is for malignancy, it would be impractical to postpone this for 3 months. The patient has good functional capacity. A cardiology opinion should be sought, and management may include stress testing and post-myocardial infarction treatment (including a beta-blocker which may also reduce peri-operative risk). Inform the anaesthetist, as the anaesthetic technique and post-operative care may be modified (see Fig. 9.6). A discussion of the risks involved should take place between the doctors involved and the patient.

3 The questions are: How significant is this patient's ischaemic heart disease? What is his peri-operative cardiac risk? Can that risk be reduced by any specific measures? 'Safe' implies negligible risk, a term which should be avoided in this situation (see Figs 9.4 and 9.5). He is an intermediate risk patient having intermediate risk surgery. You need to ascertain his functional capacity, which may be masked by his limited mobility. Cardiology referral, stress testing, peri-operative beta-blockers and modification of anaesthetic technique and post-operative care are the issues that need to be considered.

4 Management in this case starts with A (airway and oxygen), B (breathing), C (circulation) and D (disability). She requires humidified oxygen therapy, antibiotics for community acquired pneumonia and fluid challenges for volume depletion. As she is drowsy, her pupil reactions, capillary glucose and neurological examination should be recorded. She needs to be catheterised and given analgesia (not non-steroidals because of renal impairment). Full blood count, urea and electrolytes and creatinine kinase should be requested. She should be observed closely in an appropriate area and reassessed frequently by the doctor. Outcome is better after a fractured neck of femur if surgery is within 24 h. The dilemma here is that delaying surgery for too long may not help. Early surgery, post-operative care in a HDU, physiotherapy and early mobilisation may in fact be better.

5 This man has a new diagnosis of COPD. This can be confirmed by pulmonary function tests. He needs treatment for this condition under the supervision of a chest physician. Once this is done and the patient is as fit as he can be (which may mean he is still breathless and hypoxaemic), the following recommendations should be made: the patient should stop smoking, peri-operative inhaled beta-agonists should be prescribed, early mobilisation and chest physiotherapy are indicated after surgery and a discussion should take place between the anaesthetist and surgeon about the surgical and anaesthetic technique best suited to this patient.

6 The abrupt withdrawal of this patient's beta-blocker and possible electrolyte disturbance (from bowel obstruction and i.v. fluid administration) have caused AF in this lady with ischaemic heart disease. Treatment still starts with ABC. Correction of any low potassium or magnesium and i.v. administration of a rate slowing drug is a logical course of action in this case.

7 This patient is a high-risk patient as described in the pre-operative optimisation trials. He is showing signs of organ hypoperfusion and has developed acute renal failure. He is an ideal candidate for referral to a HDU or ICU for sophisticated monitoring and optimisation of cardiac output and oxygen delivery. Optimisation after surgery is less effective. Start with A (airway and oxygen), B (breathing) and C (circulation).

References

1. Royal Society. *Risk: Analysis, Perception and Management*, Report of a Royal Society study group. Royal Society, London, 1992.
2. Knaus WA, Zimmerman JE *et al*. APACHE – acute physiology and chronic health evaluation: a physiologically based classification system. *Critical Care Medicine* 1981; **9**: 591–597.
3. Wong DT and Knaus WA. Predicting outcome in critical care: the current status of the APACHE prognostic scoring system. *Canadian Journal of Anaesthesia* 1991; **38**: 374–383.
4. Copeland GP, Jones D and Walters M. POSSUM: a scoring system for surgical audit. *British Journal of Surgery* 1991; **78**: 355–360.
5. www.sfar.org/scores2/possum2.html
6. Adams AM and Smith AF. Risk perception and communication: recent developments and implications for anaesthesia. *Anaesthesia* 2001; **56**: 745–755.
7. Calman KC and Royston HD. Risk language and dialects. *British Medical Journal* 1997; **315**: 939–942.
8. Chassot P-G, Delabays A and Spahn DR. Preoperative evaluation of patients with, or at risk of, coronary artery disease undergoing non-cardiac surgery. *British Journal of Anaesthesia* 2002; **89(5)**: 747–759.
9. Grish M, Trayner E, Dammann O *et al*. Symptom-limited stair climbing as a predictor of post-operative cardiopulmonary complications after high risk surgery. *Chest* 2001; **120**: 1147–1151.
10. American College of Cardiology practice guidelines: perioperative cardiovascular evaluation for non-cardiac surgery. www.acc.org/clinical/statements.htm
11. Lee TH, Marcantonio ER, Mangione CM *et al*. Derivation and prospective validation of a simple index for prediction of cardiac risk of major non-cardiac surgery. *Circulation* 1999; **100**: 1043–1049.
12. Goldman L, Cardera DL, Nussbaum SR *et al*. Multifactorial index of cardiovascular risk in noncardiac surgical patients. *New England Journal of Medicine* 1977; **297**: 845–850.
13. Detsky AS, Abrams HB and McLauchlin JR. Predicting cardiac complications in patients undergoing noncardiac surgery. *Journal of General Internal Medicine* 1986; **1**: 211–219.
14. Poldermans D, Boersma E, Bax JJ *et al*. The effect of bisoprolol on perioperative mortality and myocardial infarction in high risk patients undergoing vascular surgery. *New England Journal of Medicine* 1999; **341**: 1789–1794.

15. Devereaux PJ, Scott Beattie W, Choi PTL *et al*. How strong is the evidence for the use of perioperative beta blockers in non-cardiac surgery? Systematic review and meta-analysis of randomised controlled trials. *British Medical Journal* 2005; **331**: 313–321.

16. Bolsin S and Colson M. Beta-blockers for patients at risk of cardiac events during non-cardiac surgery: anaesthetists should wait for better evidence of benefit. *British Medical Journal* 2005; **331**: 919–920.

17. Older P, Hall A and Hader R. Cardiopulmonary exercise testing as a screening test for peri-operative management of major surgery in the elderly. *Chest* 1999; **116**: 355–362.

18. Bland RD, Shoemaker WC, Abraham E and Cobo JC. Haemodynamic and oxygen transport patterns in surviving and non-surviving postoperative patients. *Critical Care Medicine* 1985; **13**: 85–90.

19. Shoemaker WC, Appel P, Kram HB *et al*. Prospective trial of supranormal values of survivors as therapeutic goals in high-risk surgical patients. *Chest* 1988; **94**: 1176–1186.

20. Boyd O, Grounds RM and Bennett ED. A randomised clinical trial of the effect of deliberate peri-operative increase in oxygen delivery on mortality in high-risk surgical patients. *Journal of the American Medical Association* 1993; **270**: 2699–2707.

21. Wilson J, Woods I, Fawcett J *et al*. Reducing the risk of major elective surgery: randomised control trial of pre-operative optimisation of oxygen delivery. *British Medical Journal* 1999; **318**: 1099–1103.

22. Bennett-Guerrero E. Automated detection of gastric luminal partial pressure of CO_2. *Anaesthesiology* 2000; **92**: 38–45.

Further resource

- www.cpxtesting.com

CHAPTER 10

Pain control and sedation

> **By the end of this chapter you will be able to:**
> - Understand the basic physiology of acute pain
> - Know the analgesic ladder
> - Know the anti-emetic ladder
> - Administer local anaesthesia safely
> - Understand the principles of safe sedation
> - Apply this to your clinical practice

Many patients come to hospital because they are in pain. As doctors, it is our duty to relieve suffering. However, when it comes to acute illness there are a number of physiological reasons why pain control is important. The physiological effects of severe pain include:
- Tachycardia, hypertension and increased myocardial oxygen demand
- Nausea and vomiting, ileus
- Reduced vital capacity, difficulty coughing, basal atelectasis and chest infections
- Urinary retention
- Thromboembolism.

The perception of pain is subjective and differs greatly between patients. As a simple rule of thumb, 'pain is what the patient says it is'. In adults, a common way for the doctor to assess pain and any improvement is to ask the patient to rate his pain on an imaginary scale of 0–10, with 0 meaning no pain at all and 10 the worst pain ever. This is quite useful for titrating i.v. analgesia.

Physiology of acute pain

Nociceptors are the sensory receptors for pain and are nerve endings, which exist in almost all tissues. These nerve endings are damaged or stimulated by chemical mediators and transmit signals via afferent sensory pathways to the central nervous system (dorsal horn, contralateral spinothalamic tracts, thalamus and cortex). Small myelinated A-delta fibres conduct fast pain (localised, sharp pain) and larger unmyelinated C fibres conduct slow pain (diffuse, dull pain) from the peripheries. Visceral pain is poorly localised and associated with autonomic symptoms.

The 'gate control' theory of pain describes how synaptic transmission can be modified at the dorsal horn by stimulating other afferent sensory pathways, for example rubbing or applying transcutaneous nerve stimulation (TENS).

The analgesic ladder

Fig. 10.1 shows the analgesic ladder, which is an internationally recognised guideline for the prescription of analgesia. The analgesic ladder is commonly used for post-operative patients throughout UK hospitals.

Paracetamol

Paracetamol (acetaminophen) is a weak analgesic, but it has a synergistic action and reduces the need for morphine in post-operative patients. It is a prostaglandin inhibitor, acting in the brain. Prostaglandins potentiate the action of bradykinin and other polypeptides at pain receptors. The maximum dose is 4 g in 24 h. It can be given orally, rectally or i.v. (as Perfalgan®). Side effects are rare.

Non-steroidal anti-inflammatory drugs (e.g. diclofenac)

Non-steroidal anti-inflammatory drugs (NSAIDs), such as diclofenac, are potent prostaglandin inhibitors, and the peripheral action of blocking the enzyme cyclo-oxygenase results in its anti-inflammatory properties. However, bronchospasm, gastrointestinal irritation and renal failure are side effects and NSAIDs cannot be used in certain patients for this reason. Diclofenac can be given orally, rectally or intramuscularly (i.m.).

Opioids (e.g. dihydrocodeine, tramadol)

Dihydrocodeine is a synthetic derivative of codeine, with similar pharmacological effects. It has 20% of the potency of morphine and causes less side effects. The side effects of codeine include: constipation, suppression of cough,

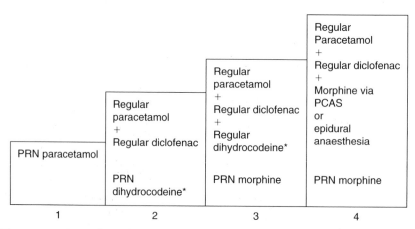

Figure 10.1 The analgesic ladder. PRN: as required; PCAS: patient controlled analgesia system. *Tramadol is an alternative opioid to dihydrocodeine.

nausea, miosis, mild sedation and confusion in the elderly. It can be given orally or i.m. Opioids are excreted by the kidneys, so the development of acute renal failure can cause accumulation and drowsiness.

Tramadol is a codeine analogue and is a weak agonist at all types of opioid receptors. It also activates descending inhibitory pain pathways. Therefore, naloxone (a pure opioid antagonist) only partly reverses the analgesic effects of tramadol. It is useful in the treatment of moderate to severe pain and can be given orally, i.m. or i.v. Tramadol reduces the seizure threshold.

Morphine

Morphine is a natural opioid and a potent analgesic. It also has sedative and anxiolytic properties. It is particularly effective for slow (C fibre) pain. Side effects, in addition to those of codeine, include respiratory depression, hypotension and histamine release (causing itching). Morphine can be given by any route. If a patient is in severe pain, there is no dose limit as long as the morphine is titrated to the pain and side effects.

Fig. 10.2 illustrates how different analgesics act at different parts of the pain pathway. Combinations of drugs can therefore be particularly effective in the treatment of pain.

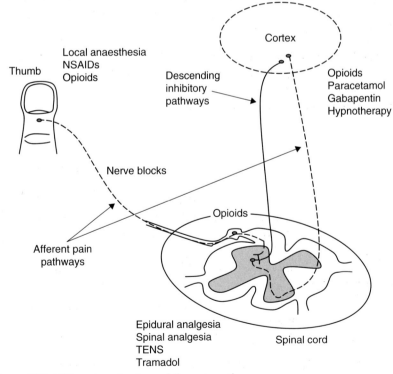

Figure 10.2 Different analgesics and the pain pathway.

When a patient presents with a serious illness and pain, titrated i.v. analgesia is the best method of pain control. This is because acute physiological stress and pain cause delayed gastric emptying, and reduced skin and muscle perfusion. Oral and i.m. analgesia may therefore be unreliable. Analgesia should be titrated to an individual's needs, rather than limited at some arbitrary level. However, sometimes pain control can be difficult. If your patient is still in pain, contact a senior doctor for help. Most UK hospitals also have an acute pain team, which is available for advice during the normal working day.

The anti-emetic ladder

Vomiting is a reflex with a sensory afferent pathway to the central nervous system. Nausea and vomiting in acute illness can be caused by stimulation of the:
• Gastrointestinal tract
• Chemoreceptor trigger zone and 'vomiting centre' in the brainstem
• Vestibular system.
Vomiting can also be caused by mechanical obstruction or ileus. Treatment of the underlying cause of nausea and vomiting is as important as symptomatic relief. The anti-emetic ladder is shown in Fig. 10.3.

Metoclopramide

Metoclopramide acts mainly by increasing gastrointestinal motility. It can cause extrapyramidal side effects and domperidone is an alternative drug, which is similar in action but does not cross the blood–brain barrier. Metoclopramide can be given orally, i.m. or i.v. It is contraindicated in intestinal obstruction.

Cyclizine and prochlorperazine

Cyclizine is an anti-histamine, used in motion sickness. It acts centrally and is slightly sedating. It can be given orally, i.m. or i.v. Prochlorperazine is a phenothiazine, many of which are used in the treatment of nausea and vomiting. Phenothiazines are potent anti-emetics, acting on the chemoreceptor trigger zone, and also have some anti-histamine, vestibular suppressant and sedative effects. Phenothiazines also cause extrapyramidal side effects. Prochlorperazine (Stemetil®) can be given orally, buccally (as Buccastem®), rectally or i.m.

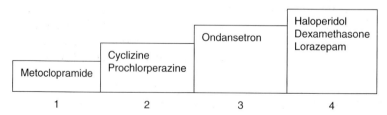

Figure 10.3 The anti-emetic ladder. In post-operative patients start at step 2.

Ondansetron

Ondansetron and Granisetron are 5-HT$_3$ receptor antagonists which act on the vagus nerve terminals. Ondansetron is used for more severe nausea and vomiting or in the post-operative period. It can be given orally, rectally, i.m. or i.v.

Haloperidol

Haloperidol is commonly used as an anti-emetic in cancer patients with problematic nausea and vomiting. It is a dopamine antagonist at the chemoreceptor trigger zone and a potent anti-emetic. Haloperidol can cause hypotension because of α blockade. It can be given orally or i.m. Extrapyramidal side effects can occur.

Dexamethasone

Dexamethasone is used for severe nausea and vomiting in cancer patients or in the post-operative period. It is a glucocorticoid with a long duration of action, so is particularly useful for delayed symptoms. It can be given orally, i.m. or i.v.

Lorazepam

Lorazepam is a benzodiazepine which is sometimes used as an anti-emetic where there is a significant anticipatory or anxiety element (e.g. following chemotherapy). It can be given orally, i.m. or i.v.

Combinations of anti-emetics which act at different sites can be particularly effective in protracted nausea and vomiting, or used prophylactically in patients known to have post-operative nausea and vomiting. Most of the anti-emetics above are also administered subcutaneously (although not licensed for this route) in palliative care situations.

Local anaesthesia

Lidocaine (formerly known as lignocaine in the UK) is the most commonly used local anaesthetic agent for practical procedures in the ward and the emergency department. It is an amide local anaesthetic and works by blocking sodium entry during depolarisation in nerve cells ('membrane stabilising'), so there is no action potential. It has a rapid onset of action and a 1% solution is effective for around 1 h. The maximum safe dose of lidocaine without epinephrine (adrenaline) is 3 mg/kg. Lidocaine is also supplied in combination with epinephrine (a potent vasoconstrictor) which prolongs its duration of action and increases the maximum dose that may be used to 7 mg/kg. Lidocaine with epinephrine is useful for suturing large scalp lacerations where there is lots of bleeding, for example. Lidocaine with epinephrine must never be used in end-extremities, and for this reason it is stored separately in UK emergency departments.

What does 1% mean? A 1% solution means there is 1 g of drug in 100 ml of solution. Put another way, there is 1000 mg of drug in 100 ml of solution, or 10 mg in 1 ml. If the maximum safe dose of lidocaine is 3 mg/kg, the maximum

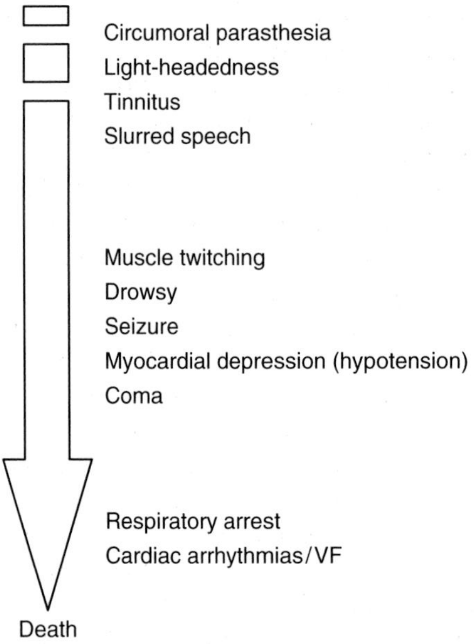

Circumoral parasthesia
Light-headedness
Tinnitus
Slurred speech

Muscle twitching
Drowsy
Seizure
Myocardial depression (hypotension)
Coma

Respiratory arrest
Cardiac arrhythmias/VF

Death

Figure 10.4 The increasing effects of lidocaine toxicity.

safe volume of lidocaine for a 70-kg man is 21 ml of 1% solution, or 10.5 ml of 2% solution. If more than the maximum recommended dose of lidocaine is used, or it is inadvertently injected i.v. (which is why you should always aspirate before injecting) toxicity may result. This is due to the 'membrane-stabilising' effect of lidocaine on the heart and central nervous system. Fig. 10.4 shows the increasing effects of lidocaine toxicity.

Treatment of lidocaine toxicity is supportive, that is ABC (oxygen and i.v. fluid). The agent is rapidly metabolised, except in liver failure or very poor hepatic blood flow (e.g. in cardiac arrest). Lidocaine should obviously *not* be given as a treatment for any arrhythmias that occur as a result of toxicity.

Other commonly used local anaesthetic agents are bupivocaine (Marcaine®), which has a slower onset and longer duration of action compared with lidocaine. The maximum safe dose is 2 mg/kg (3 mg/kg with epinephrine). Levobupivocaine is the L isomer of bupivocaine and is less toxic to the cardiovascular and nervous system. Remember that once local anaesthesia has worn off, the patient may require post-procedure analgesia.

The principles of safe sedation

Sedation is sometimes used during practical procedures to make the experience more acceptable to patients, or to make the procedure possible in an unwell agitated patient. However, the use of sedation can cause potentially life-threatening complications. There have been a number of publications on the safe use of sedation [1,2] as well as specialty specific guidelines, but also evidence that these guidelines are not followed in practice [3,4].

Sedation is defined as 'the use of a drug or drugs which produces depression of the central nervous system enabling treatment to be carried out, but during which verbal contact with the patient is maintained throughout' [5]. If this verbal contact is lost, in effect the patient is anaesthetised rather than sedated. This requires a different level of care – a separate person skilled in airway management whose only job is to monitor and care for the patient (i.e. an anaesthetist). One cannot be both the anaesthetist and the operator.

Sedation generally consists of an i.v. benzodiazepine used either alone or in combination with an opiate. The most commonly used benzodiazepines are midazolam and diazepam. Midazolam is preferred because of its quick onset of action and high amnesic qualities. It is given in small boluses (0.5–1.0 mg) titrated to effect. The dose depends on age, illness and other medication. Small doses of i.v. opiates can be given for analgesia, but should be used with caution as even small doses of such drugs can result in loss of consciousness in some patients. Drugs which depress the central nervous system also depress ventilation and have cardiovascular effects, especially in the elderly or in sick patients. Therefore, when sedation is being used, the patient should be closely monitored. A summary of the UK guidelines on safe sedation [6] is shown in Box 10.1.

Box 10.1 Guidelines on safe sedation

- The patient should be assessed beforehand for any risk factors with regard to sedation (e.g. chest and heart disease) and informed consent obtained
- A careful explanation of the procedure will help to allay anxiety and discomfort
- Obtain secure i.v. access in case of emergency
- A trained individual should monitor the patient throughout using:
  - Continuous pulse oximetry
  - Cardiac monitor
  - Regular BP readings (e.g. using an automated machine)
- Oxygen therapy reduces hypoxaemia during sedation and should be available
- Facilities must include: a bed or trolley capable of tipping head down (in case of vomiting, to prevent aspiration), a cardiac arrest trolley
- An antidote to the sedation must be immediately available (e.g. flumazenil for benzodiazepines)
- Sedation is defined as central nervous system depression while being able to maintain verbal contact. (Speaking is impossible during some procedures, e.g. bronchoscopy but the general principle applies.) If 'deep sedation' is required, an anaesthetist should be present

Treatment of benzodiazepine overdose is usually supportive. Flumazenil (Annexate) is a specific benzodiazepine antagonist which acts for about 60 min after injection. Sedation can return after this period, so the patient must be monitored for this.

Many procedures cause pain or discomfort. Analgesia should be given separately for pain, rather than more sedation. Naloxone is a specific opiate antagonist and should be available. However, it causes catecholamine release and should be used with caution in the elderly or those with ischaemic heart disease. Topical local anaesthetic sprays and infiltrative local anaesthesia are effective alternatives. A good bedside manner and proper explanation of the procedure before and during also reduces anxiety and discomfort.

Doctors who use sedation should be fully trained and responsible for ensuring that there is adequate monitoring and resuscitation facilities available.

Key points: pain control and sedation

- Pain control is an important part of acute care and has many physiological benefits.
- The analgesic ladder is used in the treatment of pain.
- The anti-emetic ladder is used in the treatment of nausea and vomiting.
- Combinations of drugs which act at different sites are particularly effective.
- The maximum safe dose of local anaesthesia should be calculated before use.
- Sedation should be administered and monitored by trained personnel.

Self-assessment: case histories

1 A 21-year-old man is admitted with viral meningitis. He complains of a severe headache and is not vomiting. There are no allergies or past medical history. What would be an appropriate analgesia prescription for this patient?

2 A 50-year-old man is admitted with an acute myocardial infarction. He complains of severe chest pain which has not improved with sublingual nitrate and oxygen. What would be an appropriate next step in terms of analgesia?

3 A 30-year-old man is about to have a chest drain inserted. He weighs 60 kg. Calculate the maximum safe dose of lidocaine and prescribe post-procedure analgesia.

4 A 60-year-old lady requires an emergency DC cardioversion for a broad complex tachycardia. You are told to give i.v. midazolam first. What do you need to consider?

5 A 25-year-old lady is extremely nauseated and vomiting following a laparascopic gynaecological procedure. Intravenous cyclizine as required is not helping. What would you prescribe next?

Self-assessment: discussion

1 Any patient admitted because of pain (e.g. severe headache) should be pre-scribed *regular* analgesia. An appropriate prescription to start with in this case would be step 2 – regular paracetamol plus diclofenac with PRN dihy-drocodeine. The patient's pain should be reviewed on a regular basis. Many patients with severe pain require a bolus of analgesia to control their pain before commencing regular 'maintenance' analgesia. Therefore, if the first dose of paracetamol, diclofenac and dihydrocodeine dose not work, an i.v. opioid, for example tramadol, could be given. Morphine tends to be avoided in meningitis and patients with brain injury because of its sedative side effects which could mask any drowsiness caused by the condition itself.

2 Intravenous morphine is used in cardiac pain because it also causes vaso-dilatation and has an anxiolytic effect. This should be drawn up in a labelled syringe containing 1 mg of morphine per ml and given by a trained mem-ber of staff (which might mean you) in small (1–2 mg) boluses until the pain is controlled. Every patient is different. He might require 2 or 20 mg of mor-phine to treat his pain. As long as the patient is still alert and complaining of pain, further small doses can be given. Ask the patient to rate his pain on a scale of 0–10 to get an idea of how effective the morphine is. Give further boluses every few minutes if pain is still present. Closely observe the patient's respiratory rate, BP and conscious level. Stop if side effects occur. Morphine causes nausea by stimulating the chemoreceptor trigger zone. An anti-emetic such as cyclizine may therefore be required.

3 The maximum safe dose of lidocaine is 3 mg/kg, or 180 mg in this case. That is 18 ml of 1% lidocaine or 9 ml of 2% lidocaine. To safely give more volume, lidocaine with epinephrine (adrenaline) can be used. The maximum safe dose would then be 7 mg/kg, or 42 ml of 1% lidocaine with epinephrine.

4 Sedation is defined as 'the use of a drug or drugs which produces depres-sion of the central nervous system enabling treatment to be carried out, but during which verbal contact with the patient is maintained throughout'. For DC cardioversion, a patient has to be unconscious. This is not sedation, this is anaesthesia. Call an anaesthetist.

5 Post-operative nausea and vomiting is common in younger women and after abdominal or gynaecological surgery. Regular cyclizine could be pre-scribed, but most anaesthetists would go to step 3 next. Ondansetron is commonly used in post-operative nausea and vomiting and is a powerful anti-emetic. It is also the anti-emetic of choice after laparoscopic surgery. It should be prescribed regularly for a while, and can also be used in combin-ation with other anti-emetic drugs.

References

1. Bell GD, McCloy RF, Charlton JE *et al*. Recommendations for standards of sedation and patient monitoring during gastrointestinal endoscopy. *Gut* 1991; **32**: 823–827.

2. Royal College of Surgeons of England. *Report of the Working Party on Guidelines for Sedation by Non-anaesthetists*, 1993.
3. Honeybourne D and Neumann CS. An audit of bronchoscopy procedures in the UK. A study of adherence to national guidelines. *Thorax* 1997; **52**: 709–713.
4. Sutaria N, Northridge D and Denvir M. A survey of current practice of transoesophageal echocardiography in the UK. Are recommended guidelines being followed? *Heart* 2000; **84(S2)**: 19.
5. Skelly AM. Analgesia and sedation. In: Watkinson A and Adam A, eds. *Interventional Radiology*. Radcliffe Medical Press, Oxford, 1996.
6. UK Academy of Medical Royal Colleges. Implementing and ensuring safe sedation practice for healthcare procedures in adults. *Report of an Intercollegiate Working Party Chaired by the Royal College of Anaesthetists*. London, 2001.

Further resource

• Whitwam JG and McCloy RF (eds). *Principles and Practice of Safe Sedation*, 2nd edn. Blackwells, Oxford, 1998.

APPENDIX
Practical procedures

By the end of this section you will be able to:
- Know the theory behind the following practical procedures
- Apply this to your clinical practice

This appendix is not intended to replace practical experience, rather to impart useful background knowledge which can then be applied under supervision. *All* of the following procedures require attention to a strict aseptic technique. This means a sterile operative field, a sterile trolley, thoroughly washed hands, sterile gloves, sterile gown and mask. Needles or lines should not be inserted through infected skin. The patient's platelet count and clotting screen should be checked before any practical procedure and the risks vs benefits should be considered and discussed.

The following practical procedures are described here:
- Lumbar puncture (LP)
- Central venous access
- Chest drain
- Abdominal paracentesis
- Pulmonary artery (PA) catheterisation.

Lumbar puncture

The first paragraphs on LP will concentrate on the practicalities of positioning the patient and the relevant anatomy. This will be followed by a section on needle size and type, and best practice to prevent and treat post-LP headache.

LP is used for:
- Obtaining sample of cerebrospinal fluid (CSF)
- Measuring CSF pressure
- Administering drugs (e.g. spinal anaesthesia).

Positioning the patient for LP

Physicians in the UK tend to perform LP with the patient lying down (left lateral position), whereas anaesthetists in the UK tend to do so with the patient sitting. There is no advantage of one technique over the other – it depends on the condition of the patient and the preference of the operator. Box A.1

Box A.1 Equipment required for LP

- Dressing pack (or LP pack)
- Extra gauze swabs
- Iodine or chlorhexadine for skin
- 10 ml 1% lignocaine
- One green needle and one blue/orange needle
- 10 ml syringe
- Sterile gloves
- Large sterile towel with window (or several sterile towels)
- Sterile gown
- Surgical mask
- At least 2 × 22G LP needles
- CSF manometer to measure pressure
- Sterile sample containers
- One large plastic backed towel to protect bed

---

shows the equipment needed to set up a trolley in preparation for an LP in the ward.

For the left lateral position, ensure the hips and shoulders are square – in line with each other and perpendicular to the bed. Then flex the spine as much as possible (foetal position) to open up the gaps between the vertebrae. The line that connects both posterior superior iliac spines (Tuffier's line) is level with L4. Midway along this line is the space between L3 and L4 which is commonly used and easily accessed. Allow time for the local anaesthetic to be effective and insert the LP needle at 90° to the skin. Aim slightly towards the umbilicus. Most operators find the right spot between spinous processes, but tend to go off track laterally, hitting other parts of the lumbar vertebra.

The sitting position is useful if the patient is obese or previous attempts in the left lateral position have failed. Put the patient's feet on a low stool with the elbows resting on the thighs. This opens up the gaps between the vertebrae. Ensure the patient is sitting straight and not leaning to one side. Fig. A.1 shows the correct positioning of a patient for LP.

The needle traverses the skin, subcutaneous tissue, supraspinous and interspinous ligaments, and ligamentum flavum before crossing the epidural space and piercing the dura with a characteristic 'pop' (see Fig. A.2). CSF pressure should always be measured if LP is being performed for diagnostic purposes. It may be the only abnormality which leads to further investigations. Normal CSF pressure in the lumbar spine is up to 18 cmH$_2$O lying or 25 cmH$_2$O sitting in adults.

Needle size and type and preventing post-LP headache

LP is commonly complicated by headache after the procedure. At least 30% of patients will suffer a post-LP headache when a 20G bevelled needle is used

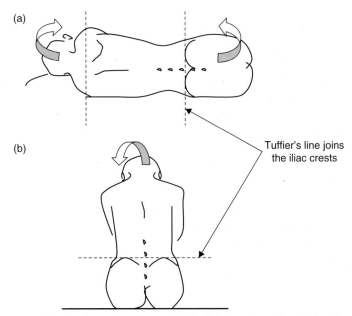

Figure A.1 Positioning the patient for LP. (a) The left lateral position is ideal for patients who are unwell and (b) the sitting position may be preferred in more difficult cases.

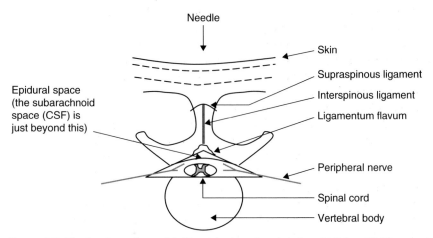

Figure A.2 The lumbar spine at L1. The spinal cord ends below L1/L2 and LP is usually performed at L3/L4.

[1], commonly found in medical wards in the UK. Young age, female sex and obstetric patients are most susceptible, hence this has been an area of extensive research in anaesthesia. Surveys have revealed that doctors who perform LPs in the ward do not use the correct needle size and type, thus increasing the risk of post-LP complications for their patients [2, 3].

Post-LP headache can be incapacitating. Rare neurological complications can also occur, such as cranial nerve palsies and subdural haematoma. It is thought that a hole is left in the dura after the LP needle has been withdrawn. This hole allows CSF to leak further, lowering CSF volume and causing discomfort through traction of the dural membranes when the patient sits up. This theory is supported by many studies that have looked at ways to try and reduce the size of the hole, by the clinical presentation of post-LP headache and by the efficacy of its treatment – extradural blood patch.

Classically, post-LP headache is related to posture (worse on sitting or standing and eased by lying down), is throbbing in nature and varies in severity. It usually presents 24–48 h after LP. The patient may be unable to mobilise because of the headache. In theory, abdominal compression can be used to confirm the diagnosis [4]. With the patient sitting and symptomatic, the waist is slowly squeezed from behind. This compresses the inferior vena cava, causes the epidural veins to become engorged and displaces CSF into the head, relieving the headache.

Although patient characteristics cannot be changed, there are four key things that the operator can do to reduce post-LP headache:
1 Use the optimum needle size
2 Use the optimum needle type
3 If using a bevelled needle, orientate it so that it faces laterally
4 Reinsert the stylet before withdrawing the needle.
Smaller needles give less risk of post-LP complications, but may not allow CSF to flow freely enough to accurately measure pressure, or may not be rigid enough for use in older people with calcified ligaments. Studies have explored which needle size gives both optimum CSF flow with the least post-LP complications [5–7]. A 22G 'atraumatic' needle is probably the best for diagnostic LPs in adults. Smaller needles are used in anaesthesia. Fig. A.3 shows the three main types of spinal needle available.

Needles with 'atraumatic' tips theoretically part, rather than cut, the elastic fibres in the dura, thus allowing them to close on withdrawal and minimising any CSF leak. If a bevelled needle is used, it should be orientated so that the bevel aligns with, rather than crosses, the dural fibres which run longitudinally.

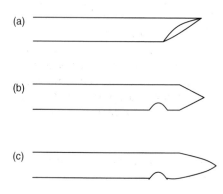

(a)

(b)

(c)

Figure A.3 Types of spinal (LP) needle. (a) Quincke (bevelled) tip with a cutting edge, (b) Whitacre and (c) Sprotte needles have atraumatic tips with the hole in the side.

Replacing the stylet before withdrawing the needle is thought to push back any strands of tissue and helps to minimise the size of the hole in the dura. Studies have shown that this manoeuvre alone significantly reduces the incidence of post-LP headache [8].

Treatment of post-LP headache

Conservative management usually works for post-LP headache: bed rest, analgesia and increased fluids. The headache often settles over a few days. However, some cases are severe. The most effective treatment is an autologous extradural blood patch; 10–20 ml of the patient's own blood is withdrawn and injected into the extradural space by an experienced anaesthetist; 90% of headaches are relieved after the first patch and up to 98% after two. This procedure literally patches up the hole in the dura.

It has become common practice to enforce bed rest following an LP (usually for 4 h). Randomised-controlled trials have not found any difference in the incidence of post-LP headache when comparing gentle mobilisation with bed rest [9]. Telling the patient to drink plenty of fluid and gently mobilise if he is able is reasonable advice.

Central venous access

The first paragraphs will describe the three main anatomical approaches used to cannulate a central vein in the neck. Then the insertion of a femoral central line is described. The Seldinger technique of inserting a central venous cannula is discussed. Finally, the use of ultrasound is described. The interpretation of central venous pressure (CVP) readings is discussed in Chapter 5.

Central lines are used for:
- Delivering irritant or vasoactive drugs
- Measurements
- Venous access.

The indications and risks should be weighed in each case before deciding to insert a central line in the neck. It is sometimes tempting to say 'this patient needs a central line' without any thought as to what it will be used for or who will measure and interpret the readings. Will it add to regular clinical assessments of the patient? A central line itself is not a treatment for anything.

Line sepsis is the most common complication of central lines and a strict sterile technique must be employed when inserting one. Immediate complications include arterial puncture, pneumothorax, damage to other surrounding structures and arrhythmias (if the wire or line enters the right atrium). A cardiac monitor should be attached to the patient during the procedure. Box A.2 shows the equipment needed to set up a trolley for a central line.

Anatomical approaches in the neck

Every doctor learning to put in a central line in the neck should first study the relevant anatomy. A basic diagram is shown in Fig. A.4. There are three main

Box A.2 Equipment required for a central line

- Suture pack
- Triple lumen central line pack (which usually includes scalpel and 5 ml syringe)
- Extra gauze swabs
- One sterile gown
- Surgical mask
- Three sterile towels
- Sterile gloves
- Iodine or chlorhexadine for skin
- 20 ml 1% lignocaine
- Two green needles and one blue/orange needle
- 10ml syringe
- 5 × 5 ml water for injections
- One size 2.0 silk suture – curved needle
- Two large clear (Tegaderm®) dressings
- One large plastic backed towel to protect bed

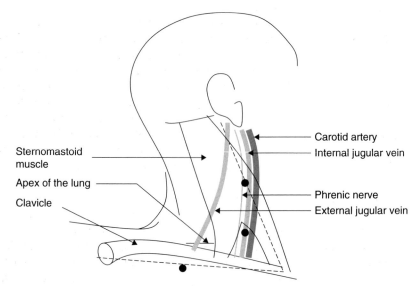

Figure A.4 Anatomy of the neck.

anatomical approaches used to cannulate a central vein in the neck, and the needle points of entry are shown in the diagram by black circles:
- Internal jugular high approach
- Internal jugular low approach
- Subclavian approach.

It is usual for the jugular vein to be cannulated on the right side, because it is aligned with the superior vena cava and right atrium more directly, and it is easier to perform for right-handed operators. The patient lays straight and flat with his head turned to the left and the bed tilted head down. This distends the vein, making it easier to cannulate, and reduces the risk of air embolism. For the high jugular approach, draw an imaginary line between the right mastoid process and the suprasternal notch. Half-way along this line is where the vein can be found, lying within the carotid sheath just lateral to the artery. Some people locate this spot by moving laterally from the cricoid cartilage. The vein is easily compressible and lies just underneath the sternomastoid muscle. A finger can palpate the carotid pulsation to ensure that the needle is directed away from it, but avoid pressing too hard as this can compress the vein. If you are not using ultrasound, locate the vein with a small 'seeker' needle first. Aim towards the right nipple at an angle of 45° to the floor. The internal jugular vein does not lie far beneath the skin unless the patient is obese. A common mistake is to insert the needle in too far, missing the vein, with the risk of damage to surrounding structures.

In the low jugular approach, the needle is inserted at the apex of the triangle formed by the two heads of sternomastoid and directed slightly laterally. A pneumothorax is more likely with this approach, although the anatomical landmarks are more reliable.

For the subclavian approach, draw an imaginary line between the acromio-clavicular joint (tip of the shoulder) and the suprasternal notch. Half-way along this line is where the needle is inserted, proceeds first underneath the clavicle and then towards the suprasternal notch. The key with the subclavian approach is never to let the needle point towards the floor, always keep it horizontal. This will avoid a pneumothorax. Subclavian lines may be less at risk of infection because of tunnelling before the line reaches the vein. The subclavian approach is contraindicated in clotting abnormalities and is avoided in patients where a pneumothorax could be catastrophic. If a patient already has a chest drain *in situ*, insert the central line on that side.

Femoral lines

Femoral central lines are commonly used in situations such as trauma and renal replacement therapy. The needle is inserted just below the inguinal ligament and medial to the femoral artery, with the hip abducted slightly. This approach is quicker and has less risk of immediate complications compared to a central line in the neck. However, line infection may be more likely. Fig. A.5 illustrates the anatomy of the femoral vein.

The Seldinger technique

The Seldinger technique is named after a Swedish radiologist who described this method of cannulating a blood vessel in the 1950s. The Seldinger technique is used for percutaneous tracheostomies, chest drains and paracentesis as well as central lines and is safer and more reliable than using a cannula-over-needle

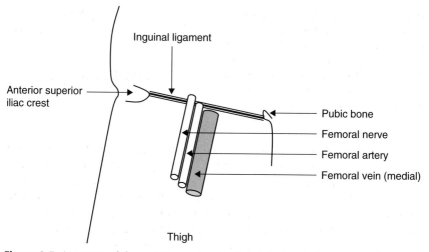

Figure A.5 Anatomy of the right femoral vein. For right-handed operators, the right femoral vein is easier to cannulate.

method. A needle is inserted into the desired space, then a wire introduced through the needle. The needle is removed and a cannula placed over the wire. Finally the wire is removed. This technique has been refined to include the use of dilators over the wire before a cannula is inserted.

Central line kits usually come with two needles. One is a cannula-over-needle (*not used*) and the other is a plain needle through which the wire passes. The wire should only be inserted as far as the catheter tip will go, as pushing it unnecessarily further can cause arrhythmias. A single dilator is used before threading the cannula over the wire. This should only be inserted far enough to open up the vessel puncture site and not pushed to its full length. These rigid dilators are manufactured longer than is necessary to allow for different anatomical approaches and patient sizes. Pushing the dilator in all the way unnecessarily can cause a haemothorax or haemopericardium and the UK's Medical Devices Agency has issued a warning to this effect [10].

A standard triple lumen central line is 20-cm long. A chest X-ray should always be performed to confirm the correct position of a CVP line and to check for pneumothorax. The line tip should sit in the superior vena cava, which is just above the aortic knuckle on a chest X-ray. This approximates to 12–15 cm at the skin in an average sized adult using the high right internal jugular approach.

Ultrasound-guided central venous access

In 2002 the National Institute for Clinical Excellence (NICE) published a report on the effectiveness of using ultrasound for central venous access. It reported that 13 randomised-controlled trials have been performed looking at central venous access comparing the landmark method with using 2D real-time

Figure A.6 2D real-time ultrasound in locating the right internal jugular vein (cross-sectional view). The orientation of the image depends on the orientation of the probe. The vein is easily compressible by gentle pressure of the probe, which distinguishes it from the artery.

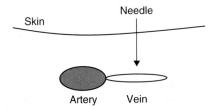

ultrasound. Outcome measures included failure rates for first and subsequent attempts, complication rates, number of needle passes and time to successful insertion. Although many of these trials were small, the evidence suggested that ultrasound guidance was significantly better than the landmark method for all outcomes for insertion into the internal jugular vein in adults. There was not enough information to comment on the subclavian approach. Ultrasound can also be used to guide the insertion of femoral lines.

The NICE guidance does concede that in an emergency the landmark method is still appropriate, and that operators experienced in the landmark method have low complication rates. But between 9% and 20% of patients have either variant anatomy (e.g. the carotid artery lies over the internal jugular vein) or thrombosed veins, making ultrasound-guided access preferable. Other studies have shown that using ultrasound for a 'quick look' followed by the land-mark method by an experienced operator makes no difference to complication rates [11].

Fig. A.6 shows the images that 2D real-time ultrasound gives when cannulating the right internal jugular vein in an adult. The steps in using ultrasound are as follows:
- Use the ultrasound probe (with gel) to locate the internal jugular vein before preparing the patient. This will allow for any change of plan in case of aberrant anatomy or a thrombosed vessel.
- The operator places ultrasound gel on the probe and carefully inserts the probe into a sterile 'condom'. Extra *sterile* gel is then added to the outside. The ultrasound images should be in view of the operator, who then locates the vein with the ultrasound probe. Remember that the orientation of the probe affects the orientation of the images.
- The ultrasound probe is held in the left hand, and the needle and syringe in the right hand. Once the vein is identified, the needle can be bounced up and down on the overlying skin and this can be seen in the ultrasound. The images should follow the needle as it is inserted towards the vein.
- The probe can be rotated by 90° to get a longitudinal view of the vein. This can confirm the placement of the wire before finishing with the ultrasound.

Chest drains

This section will describe the anatomical approach for chest drain insertion and the two main techniques will be described: Seldinger technique and blunt dissection. Finally, some safety tips regarding chest drains will be discussed.

Chest drains are used for:
- Draining air, fluid or blood from the pleural cavity
- Prevention of pneumothorax prior to positive pressure ventilation in chest trauma.

There is no evidence that large drains are superior to smaller ones, except in trauma where large bore chest drains (at least 28F) are used both to drain the thoracic cavity and monitor the rate of blood loss [12]. It is now therefore common practice to use small (12F) drains for pneumothoraces and pleural effusions, which are more comfortable and better tolerated by patients. Smaller drains are usually inserted using the Seldinger technique.

Before inserting a chest drain, it is worth pointing out that bullous lung disease can easily be confused for a pneumothorax and a collapsed lung can cause a unilateral 'whiteout' as well as a massive pleural effusion. Some patients with pre-existing lung disease may have lung which remains adherent to the chest wall (seen on X-ray) – this is a contraindication to chest drain insertion.

The equipment required to set up a trolley for chest drain insertion on the ward is listed in Box A.3. Most patients find chest drain insertion painful, even with local anaesthesia, and premedication may be necessary. The patient should be monitored throughout the procedure. Vasovagal reactions are not uncommon.

Box A.3 Equipment required for a chest drain

- Chest drain kit (e.g. 12F Seldinger chest drain)
- Suture pack
- Extra gauze swabs
- Closed drainage system (underwater seal and tubing)
- One bottle sterile water for irrigation
- Sterile gloves
- Iodine or chlorhexadine for skin
- One sterile gown +/− plastic apron
- Surgical mask
- Three sterile green towels (ones with adhesive tape are best)
- 20ml 1% lignocaine
- Two green needles and one blue/orange needle
- One 20ml syringe
- Narrow blade scalpel
- Two size 2.0 silk sutures – curved needle
- Two large dressings (Tegaderm® or Primapore®)
- Elastoplast or other adhesive tape
- One large plastic backed towel to protect bed

Anatomical approach

Before inserting a chest drain, carefully review the chest X-ray and notes, and examine the patient yourself to confirm clinically the presence of a pneumothorax or effusion. Confirm the correct side. Post-thoracotomy patients may have loculated pneumothoraces or collections and expert assistance is required.

Traditional teaching is that the site for insertion of a chest drain is the 5th intercostal space just anterior to the mid-axillary line. An alternative landmark is the triangle formed by the anterior border of latissimus dorsi, the lateral border of pectoralis major and a line at the level of the nipple in men (or the 4th intercostal space). This area avoids the internal mammary artery, muscle and breast tissue, and is illustrated in Fig. A.7. The patient should recline on the bed, slightly rotated towards the operator, sitting at an angle of 45°. The arm on the side of the drain should be placed behind his or her head. Tape may be needed to strap excess subcutaneous tissue out of the way.

Some very breathless patients are unable to recline. The drain can be inserted with the patient sitting on the edge of the bed, leaning forward with his arms outstretched across a high table.

Seldinger technique vs blunt dissection

Small (12F) Seldinger chest drains are commonly used in respiratory units and medical wards, because of patient comfort and their efficacy. A small nick is made in the skin at the correct site (just above a rib to avoid the neurovascular bundle which runs below) and a large needle is inserted. Either air or pleural fluid is aspirated and this confirms the placement. The syringe is removed and a wire placed into the space through the needle. A dilator is pushed in *just far*

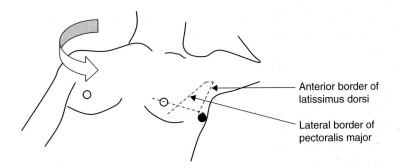

Anterior border of latissimus dorsi

Lateral border of pectoralis major

- The 'safe triangle' for insertion of a chest drain is bordered by the anterior border of latissimus dorsi, the lateral border of pectoralis major and a line at the level of the nipple (or the 4th intercostal space). The apex is just below the axilla.

- An alternative landmark is to insert the chest drain in the 5th intercostal space just anterior to the mid-axillary line (shown by the black circle).

Figure A.7 Landmarks for inserting a chest drain.

enough to create a track for the drain. The drain is threaded over the wire, then the wire is removed.

The blunt dissection technique is used for larger drains. These kits may come with a blunt introducer or a trocar. Insertion of a chest drain must *never be performed using any force* as this is dangerous. An incision just large enough for the drain is made at the correct site, just above and parallel to a rib. The operator dissects down to the pleura using forceps and eventually punctures the pleura. The drain is then inserted, using forceps to guide it. The trocar is not used.

Smaller drains tend to be curved which can help direct them towards the apex (in pneumothorax) or the base (in pleural effusion). Forceps are used to direct larger drains. A chest X-ray should be performed after the procedure to confirm the correct position.

Safety tips

Purse string sutures should not be used as they leave an unsightly scar. Secure the drain using a surgical knot. Clear dressings are easily placed over small drains so that the wound can be inspected. The drain should be tethered to the skin lower down with strong tape, so that any traction will pull here and not at the entry site.

Pleural effusions should be drained slowly as re-expansion pulmonary oedema has been described [13]. Most patients experience a mild version of this as discomfort and cough. A 3-way tap between the drain and tubing can facilitate slow drainage. The recommended rate is roughly 500 ml/h, or to clamp the tube for 1 h after 1 l has been drained. A 3-way tap should never be attached to a drain which has been inserted for a pneumothorax. This is because of the risk of accidental clamping which can lead to a tension pneumothorax. A bubbling drain should never be clamped.

Finally, patients, staff and porters all need to be educated that the underwater seal bucket should be kept upright and below the patient's waist at all times.

Abdominal paracentesis

Paracentesis means the puncture of any cavity; abdominal paracentesis refers to the drainage of ascites (for sampling or for inserting a drain). The majority of ascites in the UK is caused by liver disease, so particular attention must be paid to clotting abnormalities and platelet count before proceeding. If malignancy is suspected, an ultrasound is recommended first as malignant ascites can be loculated and the risk of puncturing the bowel is greater.

The equipment needed to set up a trolley in order to insert an ascitic drain is shown in Box A.4. This can be performed using the Seldinger or cannula-over-needle technique. Pregnancy is a contraindication and caution is required in patients with previous multiple abdominal surgery. The patient must have an empty bladder before proceeding.

Box A.4 Equipment required for abdominal paracentesis

- Paracentesis kit (Seldinger type or cannula-over-needle e.g. Bonano® catheter)
- Suture pack
- Extra gauze swabs
- Sterile gloves
- Four sterile towels (ones with adhesive tape are best)
- One sterile gown +/− plastic apron
- Iodine or chlorhexadine for skin
- 20 ml 1% lignocaine
- Two green needles and one blue/orange needle
- 10 ml syringe
- Narrow blade scalpel
- One size 2.0 silk suture – curved needle
- Two large Primapore® dressings
- One large (urinary) catheter bag and stand
- One large plastic backed towel to protect bed

Anatomical approaches

The patient should lie almost flat. Before inserting an ascitic drain, carefully review the notes and examine the patient yourself to confirm clinically the presence of ascites. A midline approach is described, through the avascular linea alba just below the umbilicus, but this is not commonly used in the UK. The flank on either side is preferred, in an area of dullness to percussion, laterally enough to avoid the deep inferior epigastric artery and vein which supply the rectus muscle on either side. The right or left flank is acceptable, and may depend on individual patient characteristics (e.g. use the left flank in hepatomegaly). The correct insertion sites are shown by the black circles in Fig. A.8.

The operator should check that ascites is freely aspirated at the chosen site before inserting the drain. Some people recommend pulling the skin 1–2 in. to one side as the drain is passed through the skin and subcutaneous tissue in order to create an oblique track which minimises leakage after the drain is pulled out. Either way, leakage is common following removal of an ascitic drain and a deep suture should be placed through the hole after removal to prevent this.

Finally, if the ascites is due to portal hypertension and your centre uses human albumin solution (HAS) for this procedure, make sure that this is ordered and ready before starting. Every 2.5 l of ascites drained requires 500 ml of i.v. 4.5% HAS. Theoretically, any colloid will do for volume resuscitation in this situation. Removal of a large volume of ascites relieves the splinting effect of the fluid on intra-abdominal blood vessels and fluid shifts also occur. This can precipitate intravascular volume depletion and hypotension. BP should

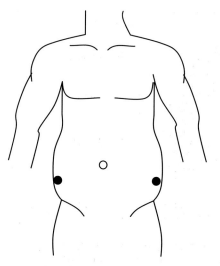

Figure A.8 Insertion sites for an ascitic tap or drain. Insertion sites are shown by the black circles.

therefore be monitored closely. The drain should always be removed 12–24 h later in order to minimise the risk of infection.

Pulmonary artery catheters

Pulmonary artery (PA), or Swan–Ganz, catheters have been used in an attempt to measure left heart pressures more directly than the CVP line, but there are still several limitations. PA catheters are used for:
- Monitoring the effects of therapy in septic shock
- Optimising therapy in situations where right atrial pressures do not reflect left heart function (e.g. cardiogenic shock)
- Pre-optimisation before major surgery
- Infusion of drugs into the pulmonary circulation (e.g. prostacyclin).

PA catheters can measure:
- CVP
- Right atrial and right ventricular pressures
- Pulmonary artery occlusion pressure (PAOP)
- Mixed venous oxygen saturation
- Cardiac output (CO)
- Systemic vascular resistance (SVR), a derived measurement.

There is no evidence that using a PA catheter improves outcome and a number of less invasive alternative techniques are becoming more common. However, the PA catheter is still used in certain settings (e.g. intensive care unit (ICU), coronary care units and during cardiac surgery) and therefore is described here. As with all haemodynamic monitors, it is important that data is always interpreted in the light of a clinical assessment of the patient.

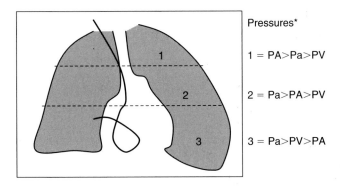

Pressures*

1 = PA>Pa>PV

2 = Pa>PA>PV

3 = Pa>PV>PA

- The catheter curls in the right ventricle and the tip sits in the pulmonary artery (lungs) but it is trying to measure pressure changes in the left ventricle – via the whole of the lungs, left atrium and mitral valve.
- The PA catheter tip must sit in a West-zone 3 of the lung. West described physiological lung zones; zone 3 is where pulmonary venous pressure is greater than alveolar pressure. If the tip is in a non-zone 3, the wedge pressure may reflect alveolar rather than left atrial pressure. Luckily, balloon catheters tend to enter zone 3 because it is the area with highest blood flow. Although West zones are anatomical in normal lungs, they are actually physiological zones which can be altered by disease. Absence of a normal waveform, a wedge pressure that fluctuates widely with respiration or a rise in wedge pressure greater than half of any PEEP increase are clues to a non-zone 3 placement.

Figure A.9 PA catheter appearance on a chest X-ray. *Pressure in the pulmonary arteries (Pa), alveolus (PA) and veins (PV).

The balloon-tipped PA catheter is 70 cm long, with markings for every 10 cm. The catheter has several channels for infusions, inflating the balloon and connections to a thermistor. Complications of the PA catheter, in addition to those of the CVP line, include:

- Transient arrhythmias, for example ventricular tachycardia (sustained arrhythmias are uncommon)
- Catheter knotting
- Damage to valves or myocardium (e.g. mural thrombus)
- Pulmonary infarction
- Pulmonary artery rupture
- Incorrect measurement and interpretation of data.

An introducer is inserted into the right internal jugular or left subclavian vein. After preparing the catheter, it is connected to a pressure transducer. The catheter is inserted to 20 cm, beyond the length of the introducer, in the large veins. The balloon is then inflated and the catheter inserted further. The balloon helps the catheter tip move with blood flow to the correct position, illustrated in Fig. A.9 – hence the expression 'floating' a PA catheter.

When the catheter tip is wedged, it directly communicates with the left atrium via the pulmonary vessels. Fig. A.10 illustrates the PA catheter trace patterns. The PAOP is approximately the same as left atrial pressure. At end diastole,

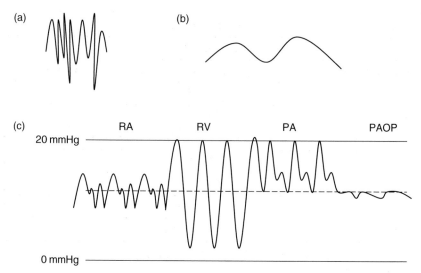

Figure A.10 PA catheter trace patterns. (a) Waving the catheter tip in mid-air before insertion produces a trace like this. (b) Air bubbles damp the trace as on the right-hand side and should be flushed out. (c) First a characteristic CVP trace is seen, followed by a right ventricular trace as soon as the catheter tip enters the right ventricle (note the higher pressures). When the catheter tip enters the pulmonary artery, the diastolic pressure increases and the trace changes to have a dichotic notch. When the balloon wedges, a damped trace is seen. The catheter must not be left wedged as pulmonary infarction may occur – this is for measurements only. In a healthy unventilated patient CVP = PAOP; RA: right atrium; RV: right ventricle.

left atrial pressure approximates to left ventricular pressure, which in turn is assumed to reflect left ventricular end-diastolic volume. Readings are taken at end expiration when intrathoracic pressure is nearest to zero. Lung and mitral valve disease are two major factors which affect the assumption that PAOP is equivalent to left ventricular end-diastolic volume. Pulmonary vascular resistance is increased in mitral stenosis, hypoxaemia, acidosis, pulmonary embolism and acute respiratory distress syndrome (ARDS). A stiff left ventricle alters the relationship between pressure and volume. Furthermore, many values from the PA catheter are derived and even entering the incorrect weight and height of the patient can introduce error.

Trends are more important than a single reading and should be used in conjunction with a thorough clinical assessment. Clinical assessment still remains far more important than numbers alone. The normal PA catheter values are shown in Fig. A.11.

CO is measured by the thermodilution method. Cold fluid is injected rapidly via the proximal PA catheter lumen into the right atrium at end expiration. The thermistor measures the temperature change downstream and a computer calculates the CO using the indicator dilution equation.

Value	Normal range
CVP	0–10 mmHg
Right ventricle	0–10 mmHg diastolic, 15–30 mmHg systolic
PAOP	5–15 mmHg
Left atrium	4–12 mmHg
Left ventricle	4–12 mmHg diastolic, 90–140 mmHg systolic
Stroke volume	55–100 ml
CO	4–8 l/min
CI	1.5–4 l/min/m^2
SVR	770–1500 dyn s/cm^5

Figure A.11 Normal PA catheter values and intra-cardiac pressures in an unventilated patient.

The PA catheter has been used to optimise CO and oxygen delivery, because it can measure CO and mixed venous oxygen saturation. The derived measurement of SVR is useful in titrating therapy in septic shock, where abnormal vasodilatation and sometimes depressed cardiac function lead to severe hypotension. PA catheters are indicated when there is an operator experienced in their use and the risk:benefit ratio to the patient is acceptable.

Key points: practical procedures

- All of the above procedures require attention to a strict aseptic technique. This means a sterile operative field, a sterile trolley, thoroughly washed hands, sterile gloves, sterile gown and mask.
- The risks vs benefits for any procedure should be considered and discussed.
- Theoretical knowledge is not the same as competence.

Self-assessment: case histories

1 A 60-year-old man is admitted to the ICU for pre-operative optimisation 6 h before a laparotomy for bowel obstruction. He is normally treated for hypertensive heart failure, which is controlled. He has developed signs of sepsis. He has warm, dry peripheries and his vital signs are: alert, pulse 98/min, BP 110/70 mmHg, respiratory rate 24/min, SpO$_2$ 95% on air, temperature

37.5°C. He says he is thirsty. His chest is clear. His PA catheter readings are as follows:

CVP = 13 mmHg
PAOP = 10 (5–15 mmHg)
CO = 5.5 (4–8 l/min)
CI = 3 (1.5–4 l/min/m^2)
SVR = 1100 (770–1500 dyn s/cm^5)

How would you treat this patient?

2 A 40-year-old man is admitted to ICU with hypotension causing hypoperfusion that has not responded to fluid challenges. He has a PA catheter inserted and the initial readings show:

CVP = 3 mmHg
PAOP = 5 (5–15 mmHg)
CO = 10 (4–8 l/min)
CI = 4.5 (1.5–4 l/min/m^2)
SVR = 300 (770–1500 dyn s/cm^5)

What diagnosis are these readings consistent with? What is your management?

Self-assessment: discussion

1 Management always starts with A (airway and oxygen), B (breathing) and C (circulation). Ignore the PA catheter readings and perform a clinical bed-side assessment. What is your clinical impression of the patient? The history points towards volume depletion. He is thirsty, with an increased respiratory rate and tachycardic. What is his normal BP? Are there any other signs of hypoperfusion (see Fig. 5.6)? If you did not have these PA catheter readings, you would give a fluid challenge and assess the response. It may be that this patient's PA catheter readings are within normal limits because he has an inadequate response to sepsis due to his heart failure. This is an example of the potential to rely on numbers rather than a clinical assessment.

2 These readings show low filling pressures (CVP and PAOP), a high CO and a low SVR. This is typical of severe sepsis. Fluid challenges should be given to optimise preload and then vasopressors added to increase SVR in order to improve tissue perfusion. Further details on the treatment of severe sepsis are given in Chapter 6.

References

1. Kuntz KM, Kokmen E, Stevens JC *et al*. Post lumbar puncture headaches: experience in 501 consecutive procedures. *Neurology* 1992; **42**: 1884–1887.

2. Broadley SA and Fuller GN. Audit of LP practice in UK neurology centres. *Journal of Neurology Neurosurgery and Psychiatry* 1997; **63**: 266.

3. Broadley SA and Fuller GN. Lumbar puncture needn't be a headache [editorial]. *British Medical Journal* 1997; **316**: 1324–1325.

4. Reynolds F. Dural puncture and headache – avoid the first but treat the second. *British Medical Journal* 1993; **306**: 874–876.

5. Kleyweg RP, Hertzberger LI and Carbaat PA. Significant reduction in post lumbar puncture headache using an atraumatic needle. A double blind controlled clinical trial. *Cephalalgia* 1998; **18(9)**: 6355–6357.

6. Braune HJ and Huffman G. A prospective double blind clinical trial comparing the sharp Quincke needle (22G) with an 'atraumatic' needle (22G) in the induction of post lumbar puncture headache. *Acta Neurologica Scandinavica* 1992; **86**: 50–54.

7. Carson D and Serpell M. Choosing the best needle for diagnostic lumbar puncture. *Neurology* 1996; **47**: 33–37.

8. Strupp M, Brandt T and Muller A. Incidence of post lumbar puncture syndrome reduced by reinserting the stylet: a randomised prospective study of 600 patients. *Journal of Neurology* 1998; **245**: 589–592.

9. Spriggs DA, Burn DJ, French J, Cartilidge NEF and Bates D. Is bed rest useful after diagnostic lumbar puncture? *Postgraduate Medical Journal* 1992; **68**: 581–583.

10. Medical Devices Agency (Department of Health). Safety warning – MDA/2003/020 – central venous catheters, dilators and guidewires. www.medical-devices.gov.uk

11. National Institute of Clinical Excellence. The effectiveness and cost-effectiveness of ultrasound locating devices for central venous access. January 2002. www.nice.org.uk

12. Lowe D, Neville E, Duffy J, on behalf of the British Thoracic Society. BTS Guidelines for the insertion of a chest drain. *Thorax* 2003; **58(S ll)**: ii53–ii59.

13. Mafhood S, Hix WR, Aaron BL *et al*. Re-expansion pulmonary oedema. Annals of Thoracic Surgery 1988; **45**: 340–345.

Index

Note: Entries taken from the figures and tables are denoted by *italicised* page numbers.